FIRST AID

St. John Ambulance Saint-Jean

SAVING LIVES
at work, home and play

SAUVER DES VIES
au travail, à la maison et dans les loisirs

REFERENCE GUIDE
Third Edition

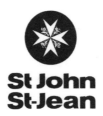

**St John
St-Jean**

Third edition – May 2018

Certification

Knowledge of the information contained in this book does not constitute an endorsement of a user's qualifications by St. John Ambulance. A user's qualifications are recognized by St. John Ambulance only after the successful completion of a St. John Ambulance training course, which includes practical activities and formal assessment of knowledge and skills, and the issuance of a training certificate.

Library and Archives Canada Cataloguing in Publication

First Aid: Reference Guide, formerly published as First on the scene: the complete guide to first aid and CPR. — 4th ed.

Includes index.

ISBN 978-1-897513-00-2

1. First aid in illness and injury. 2. CPR (First aid). I. St. John Ambulance

II. Title: First Aid : First on the Scene.

RC86.8.F59 2006 616.02'52 C2006-901819-7

Chain of Survival® is a registered trademark of the Heart and Stroke Foundation of Canada

EpiPen® Auto-Injector is a registered trademark of the EM Industries, Inc.

Tylenol® is a registered trademark of McNeil Consumer Products.

Tempra® is a registered trademark of Mead Johnson Canada.

Water-Jel® is a registered trademark of Water-Jel Technologies Inc.

Viagra® is a registered trademark of Pfizer Pharmaceuticals.

Printed in Canada   sja.ca   Stock No. 6504-16

St. John Ambulance

St. John Ambulance is a charity and international humanitarian organization dedicated to helping Canadians improve their health, safety and quality of life through training and community service. Revenue generated from first aid/CPR training supports St. John Ambulance's charitable work in Canada and around the world.

Coast-to-coast, more than 12,000 front-line volunteers serve communities by providing first aid services at public events and during emergencies. St. John Ambulance volunteers also improve quality of life through programs that help seniors, the disadvantaged, and youth.

As Canada's leading authority in first aid and CPR services since 1883, St. John Ambulance offers innovative programs and products to save lives at work, home, and play.

To contact your local St. John Ambulance, visit www.sja.ca.

Fast facts

- Established in 1883 in Canada with roots going back 900 years
- Issues over 500,000 certificates in first aid and CPR to Canadians each year
- Supports humanitarian relief efforts across Canada and around the world
- St. John Ambulance front-line volunteers provide service at approximately 10,000 public events annually
- More than 1 million volunteer hours of community service are provided annually
- More than 100,000 individuals were assisted by St. John Ambulance volunteers in 2014
- 365 Canadians were formally recognized for their efforts to save a life in 2015
- Approximately 3,000 St. John Therapy Dog teams provided over 200,000 volunteer hours in 2014

This Reference Guide was developed in accordance with the 2016 Canadian Consensus Guidelines on First Aid and CPR, an evidence-based set of recommendations on training and standards of practice for first aid and CPR. The guidelines are released by the Canadian Guidelines Consensus Task Force comprised of the Heart and Stroke Foundation, the Canadian Red Cross, St. John Ambulance, the Canadian Ski Patrol, and the Lifesaving Society.

Disclaimer

The information ("Information") provided in this book is for general use and knowledge and does not contain all information that may be relevant to every situation. The Information cannot be relied upon as a substitute for seeking guidance from appropriate professionals, such as physicians. Users acknowledge and agree that St. John Ambulance is not responsible or liable for the user's actions or decisions resulting from the information (including information regarding medication or other drugs) in this book, including but not limited to choosing to seek or not to seek advice from medical professionals such as physicians.

St. John Ambulance cautions users of this book not to prescribe or administer any medication, including over-the-counter medication, except in instances where permitted by law. Inclusion of symptom relief medication in workplace first aid kits falls outside the scope of this book. Access and dispensing of symptom relief medication in the workplace must be done in accordance with the employer directives and any applicable law.

Although St. John Ambulance takes great care to reflect the most current and accurate information at time of publication, it does not represent or warrant that the information contained in this book will be accurate or appropriate at time of reading or use due to evolving medical research, protocols, regulations and laws. It is the responsibility of the user of this book to be knowledgeable of changes in acceptable practices when providing first aid, and applicable laws and regulations in which first aid may be provided.

The information in this book is provided "as is" and without warranties or conditions of any kind either express or implied. To the fullest extent permitted by applicable law, under no circumstances, including, but not limited to, negligence, shall St. John Ambulance be liable for any direct, indirect, incidental, special or consequential damages that result in any manner from the use of or reliance on information and answers provided in this book.

Emergency Phone Numbers

	_____
Police	_____
Fire	_____
Ambulance	_____
Poison Control	_____
Emergency Contact	
Name	_____
Phone	_____
Home Phone	_____
Street Address	_____

Table of Content

Chapter 1

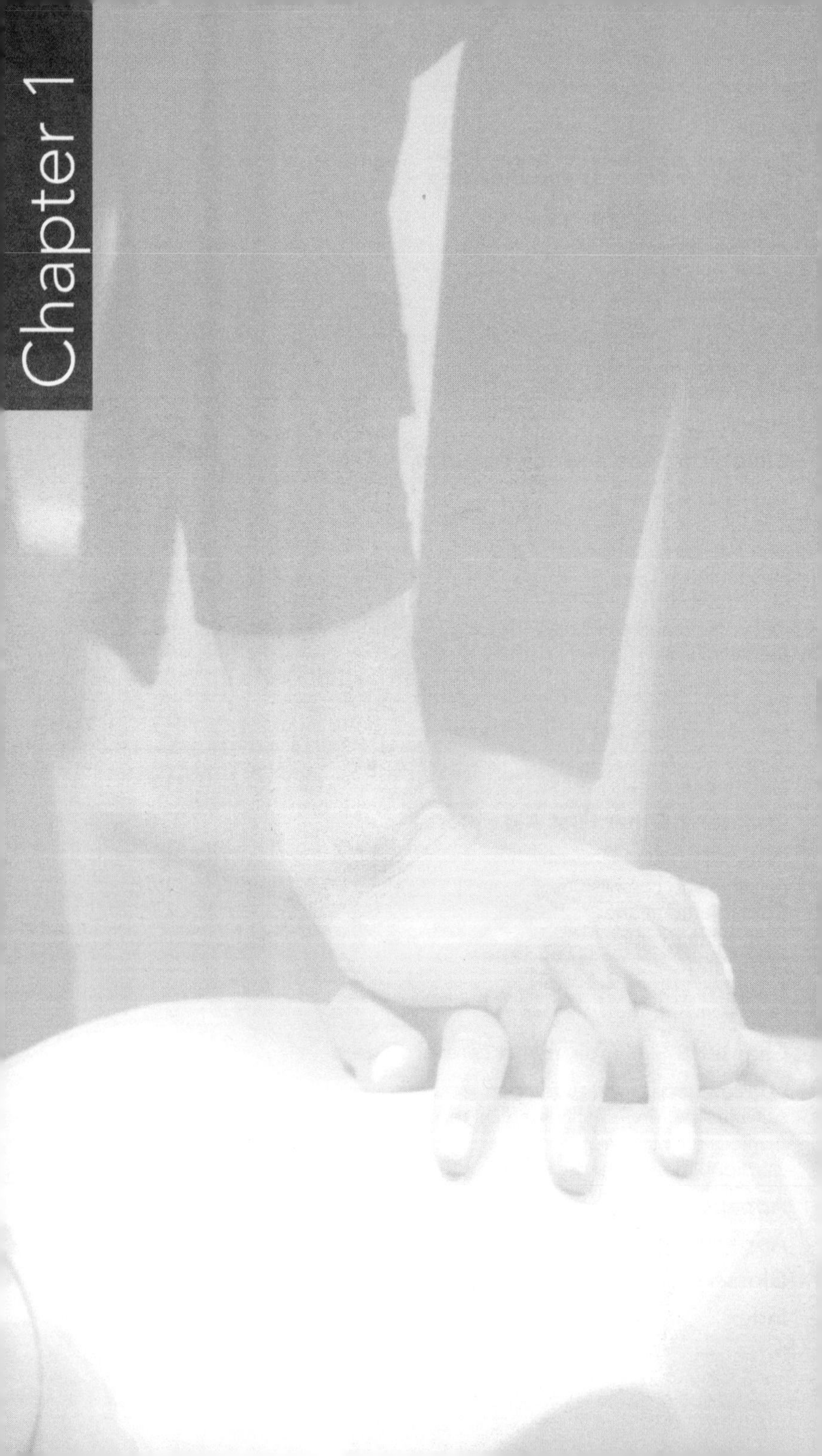

Introduction to
First Aid

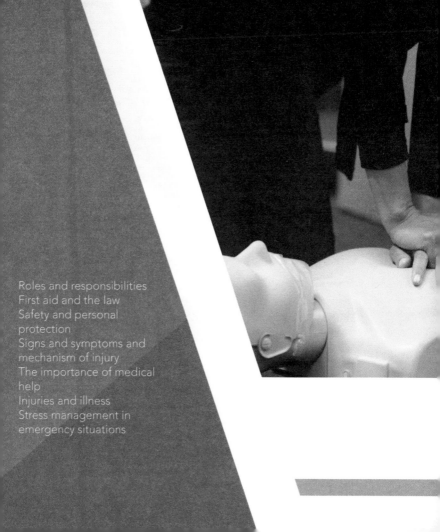

Roles and responsibilities
First aid and the law
Safety and personal
protection
Signs and symptoms and
mechanism of injury
The importance of medical
help
Injuries and illness
Stress management in
emergency situations

Chapter 1 Introduction to First Aid

This guide covers a wide range of information that will help you respond appropriately in a first aid or medical emergency. The introductory chapter contains background information, definitions and other material related to giving first aid. Chapter 2 explains casualty management including issues that relate to assessment of the casualty. This chapter also includes topics that are important to understand in the first critical moments at the emergency scene. Chapter 5 deals with issues of particular interest to health care providers—responders with a specific duty to respond within the health care system.

Roles and responsibilities

What is first aid?

First aid is emergency help given to an injured or suddenly ill person using readily available materials. A person who takes charge of an emergency scene and gives first aid is called a first aider. The injured or ill person is called a casualty.

The three priorities of first aid, in order of importance, are to:

- preserve life
- prevent the illness or injury from becoming worse
- promote recovery

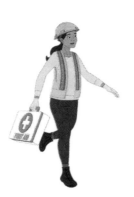
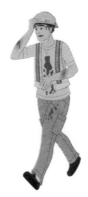

What can a first aider do?

First aiders do not *diagnose* or *treat* injuries and illnesses (except, perhaps, when they are very minor)—this is what medical doctors do. A first aider *suspects* injuries and illnesses, and gives *first aid* at the scene.

Besides giving first aid, it is important to:

- protect the casualty's belongings
- keep unnecessary people away
- reassure family or friends of the casualty
- clean up the emergency scene and work to correct any unsafe conditions that may have caused the injuries in the first place

A casualty's age in first aid and CPR

The procedures related to the provision of first aid and cardiopulmonary resuscitation (CPR) differ in some ways, depending on the age and size of the casualty.

In first aid and CPR:

- an **infant** casualty is under one year old
- a **child** casualty is from age one to age eight
- an **adult** casualty is over eight years of age

It is important to recognize that these ages are guidelines. The size of the casualty must be considered.

1

First aid and the law

Note that St. John Ambulance is not giving legal advice. This guide is not intended to replace advice given by a lawyer or legal professional.

Giving first aid as part of your job

When giving first aid is part of your job you have a duty to use reasonable skill and care based on your level of training. There are regulations to protect the first aider. For example in workplaces regulated by the Canada Labour Code, Section 126 (3) of the Code states:

"No employee is personally liable for anything done or omitted to be done in good faith by the employee when the employee is assisting the employer, as requested by the employer, in providing first-aid or in carrying out any other emergency measures."

Principles of the Good Samaritan

Across Canada Good Samaritan laws and principles protect first aiders from lawsuits. You are a Good Samaritan if you are a bystander who helps a person when you have no legal duty to do so. As a Good Samaritan, you give your help without being paid, and you give it in good faith. Whenever you help a person in an emergency situation, you should abide by the following principles:

- you identify yourself as a first aider and get permission to help the injured or ill person before you touch them—this is called **consent**

- you use **reasonable skill and care** in accordance with the level of knowledge and skill that you have

- you are not **negligent** in what you do

- you do not **abandon** the person

Consent

The law says everyone has the right not to be touched by others. As a first aider, you must respect this right.

Always ask if you can help. If the casualty cannot answer you, you have what is called **implied consent,** and you can help.

If the casualty is an infant or a young child, you must get consent from the child's parent or guardian. If there is no parent or guardian at the scene, the law assumes the casualty would give consent if they could, so you have implied consent to help.

A person has the right to refuse your offer of help. In this case, do not force first aid on a conscious casualty. If you do not have consent to help, there may be other actions you can take without touching the casualty, such as controlling the scene, and calling for medical help.

Be aware of difficulties in communicating when a casualty:

- is hard of hearing
- speaks a different language
- is visually impaired
- is a child
- is in pain
- shows signs of mood disorder

Reasonable skill and care

As a Good Samaritan, when you give first aid you are expected to use reasonable skill and care according to your level of knowledge and skills.

Negligence

Give only the care that you have been trained to provide, and always act in the best interest of the casualty.

1

Abandonment

Never abandon a casualty in your care. Stay until:

- you hand them over to medical help

- you hand them over to another first aider

- they no longer want your help—this is usually because the problem is no longer an emergency, and further care is not needed

Giving first aid in Quebec

The Quebec Charter of Human Rights and Freedoms declares that any person whose life is in danger has the right to be helped. This means that you are required to help a person whose life is at risk, provided you do not put your own life, or anyone else's, in danger.

Safety and personal protection

Always give first aid safely. There are three basic types of risks to be aware of:

- The energy source that caused the original injury—is the mechanism that caused the original injury still active, causing injury to others? Example: where an injury has been caused by machinery, is the machinery still running?

- There may be hazards caused by external factors. Example: passing vehicles may pose a risk at the scene of a motor vehicle incident

- There may be hazards associated with first aid procedures or a rescue. Example: moving a heavy casualty could place the first aider at risk of injury

Preventing infection

Airborne pathogens

Examples of infections that can be spread through the air are:

- **Meningitis** is a bacterial or viral infection which causes swelling that affects the spinal cord and brain
- **Tuberculosis** is a bacterial infection that primarily affects the lungs, but can affect any part of the body
- **Influenza**, or "the flu," is a viral infection which is easily spread, and can vary from being mildly debilitating to fatal

Body fluid and blood-borne pathogens

Exposure to blood or body fluids (i.e. vomit, feces) poses a health risk to first aiders. There are three diseases that first aiders should be aware of:

- **Human immunodeficiency virus (HIV)** is the virus responsible for AIDS. There is no vaccine to protect people from this virus. The best defence remains adequate protection to help prevent infection.
- **Hepatitis B** is one of the three common forms of hepatitis, a viral disease that can cause severe liver damage. Some people who have Hepatitis B have no symptoms but are still contagious. There is a vaccine to prevent Hepatitis B.
- **Hepatitis C** causes much of the same liver damage as Hepatitis B, but there is currently no vaccine available to prevent this disease.

Sharp objects

If a sharp object touches infected blood and then pricks or cuts you, you could become infected. First aiders do not use sharp objects like scalpels and needles, but there may be broken glass or other sharp objects that have been in contact with blood or other bodily fluids. Always wear gloves and handle sharp objects with extreme care.

1

Personal Protective Equipment

Personal Protective Equipment (PPE) is clothing and equipment used to protect the first aider and to minimize the risks of health and safety hazards when in contact with a casualty. PPE can be gloves, a pocket mask used for ventilations, a helmet, eye protection, safety boots, etc.

Use a face mask or shield when providing artificial respiration or CPR. Always follow the manufacturer's directions for disinfecting and cleaning reusable items. Single-use masks, one-way valves, and gloves are disposed of by double bagging with other contaminated articles. If used in the workplace, follow provincial/territorial and/or company protocols for disposal of hazardous items.

Disposable gloves prevent direct hand contact aider and the casualty. Wear gloves when you might touch blood, bodily fluids, tissue or anything that has come in contact with one of these.

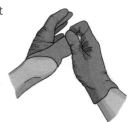

If you tear a glove, wash your hands as soon as possible, and put on a new pair. Dispose of contaminated gloves by sealing them in a plastic bag and double-bagging them.

Protecting the first aider

Areas of the body that may have come into contact with a casualty need to be cleaned with hot, soapy water, an anti-septic solution, or a mixture of bleach and water (at a ratio of 1:10). Spills should be cleaned, then sanitized with the bleach and water solution for 20 minutes.

Anyone who has been exposed to possible contaminants should take a hot shower with soap and rinse thoroughly. Anyone who has been exposed to contaminants from a needle stick or sharps injury should seek medical attention.

How to remove gloves

Once gloves have been used, they are contaminated and are a possible source of infection. Take them off without touching their outer surface following the steps below.

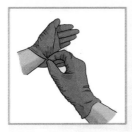

Grasp the cuff of one glove.

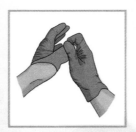

Pull the cuff towards the fingers, turning the glove inside out.

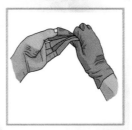

As the glove comes off, hold it in the palm of your other hand.

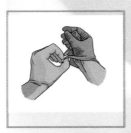

Slide your fingers under the cuff of the other glove.

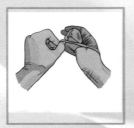

Pull the cuff towards the fingers over the first glove.

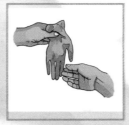

Tie a knot in the top of the outer glove and dispose of properly—see below.

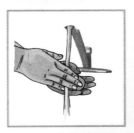

Wash hands with soap and running water as soon as possible.

Proper disposal

Seal the used gloves in a plastic bag and put them in your household garbage.

Check with a health professional or your first aid instructor for specific regulations in your area.

Help at the emergency scene

1

Bystanders should be asked to leave unless asked to stay and assist.

Other first aiders may offer to help. Identify yourself and accept their assistance. If someone is more qualified to handle the situation, you may ask that person to take control.

First responders include ambulance personnel, police officers and firefighters. They will take charge of the scene as soon as they arrive.

Other authorities may be called to the scene (e.g. an electrical utility crew may arrive if there are downed power lines). Identify yourself and continue giving first aid.

Off-duty doctors, nurses and other health professionals may identify themselves and offer to help.

If an injury occurs due to violence, or a first aider and/or casualty becomes at risk due to violence, you must protect yourself and call for help. Your skills as a first aider are valuable only when the area is safe.

Ten ways a bystander can help

1.   Make the area safe
2.   Find all the casualties
3.   Find a first aid kit
4.   Control the crowd
5.   Call for medical help
6.   Help give first aid, under your direction
7.   Gather and protect the casualty's belongings
8.   Take notes
9.   Reassure the casualty's relatives
10.   Lead the paramedics to the scene of the emergency

Signs and symptoms and mechanism of injury

When referring to injuries, first aiders need to understand **signs and symptoms.**

- A **sign** is something we can see, feel, hear or smell (e.g. bleeding, bruising, agonal breathing, skin discoloration).

- A **symptom** is something the casualty is feeling (e.g. nauseous, weakness, pain) and must tell you.

Mechanism of injury encompasses both what happened to the casualty, and how the injury has affected the casualty. It identifies the cause of the injury. Mechanisms of injury that require an ambulance right away:

- A fall from 6.5 meters (20 feet) or more

- A vehicle collision with signs of a severe impact

- Severe damage to the inside of the vehicle, a bent steering wheel, or a broken windshield

- Casualty was thrown from a vehicle

- The vehicle has rolled over

- Casualty was struck by a vehicle

- Crush injuries

When any of these mechanisms are apparent, call an ambulance as soon as you can. When we understand the cause of the injury, we are able to predict what injuries may be present and what injuries are not likely, even in situations in which there are no visible signs of injury and/or the casualty is unable to describe their symptoms.

Signs and symptoms

1

Examples of Signs and Symptoms	
signs you can see	blood, deformity, bruising, unequal pupils, painful expression and/or flinching, sweating, wounds, unusual chest movement, skin colour, swelling, foreign bodies, vomit, incontinence
signs you can hear	noisy or distressed breathing, groans, sucking wounds (chest injury), bones scraping together, quality of speech
signs you can feel	dampness, skin temperature, swelling, deformity
signs you can smell	casualty's breath (fruity breath, acetone/nail polish breath, or alcohol), vomit, incontinence, gas fumes, burning, solvents or glue
symptoms the casualty may tell you about	pain, fear, heat, cold, loss of normal movement, loss of sensation, numbness, tingling sensation, thirst, nausea, faintness, stiffness, feeling faint, weakness, memory loss, dizziness, sensation of a broken bone

The importance of medical help

1

In first aid, any type of medical care is referred to as medical help. Unless an injury is very minor, you should always make sure the casualty receives medical help following first aid. Medical help may be given at the scene, en route to a medical facility, or in a hospital.

Know the EMS telephone number for your community. This is often 9-1-1 in urban areas. If you are outside of your community, find the EMS phone numbers in the first few pages of the telephone book, or search online.

Calling for medical help is important. The period immediately following a severe, life-threatening injury is known as the **golden hour**. This time is "golden" because the faster a casualty makes it to a hospital emergency room or operating room, the better the chances of survival and recovery.

You can ask a bystander to call for medical help. Provide the person with:

• Necessary phone number

• A description of the casualty's condition

• Directions to follow to reach the scene

• Instructions to report back to you after getting medical help

If you are alone, you must decide whether to stay with the casualty or leave to get help. The correct decision will depend on the specifics of the situation. If you have a mobile phone, call from the scene and perform first aid with the dispatcher's assistance.

Medical care

1

As a first aider you are not trained to diagnose the nature and extent of an injury or illness; a medical doctor has the training to do this. As a rule, make sure the casualty receives medical care following first aid. For minor injuries, this may not be necessary. **Medical care** is either given by a medical doctor or under the supervision of a medical doctor. Paramedics give medical care because they work under the supervision of medical doctors. Medical care is given in hospitals but it can also be given at the emergency scene or on the way to a medical facility.

Call an ambulance or drive the casualty to the hospital?

Always call an ambulance if you can; only transport the casualty to medical help yourself if that is the only possible way to get medical help. Transporting an injured person is often difficult and time-consuming. An ambulance or other rescue vehicle is well-equipped, and the casualty can begin receiving medical help as soon as it arrives.

The Good Samaritan principles only protect you when giving care at the scene of the emergency, or while transporting the casualty when this is needed to save the casualty's life and medical help is not available. Transporting the casualty unnecessarily leaves you liable if it results in further injury should an accident or incident occur while en route to a hospital or medical station.

Good communication

1

Communication is necessary in every emergency situation, regardless of the details. As the first aider, there are many people you may need to communicate with – the casualty, bystanders, family members, other first aiders, EMS providers, and other professionals (e.g. police, fire, hydro). Effective communication skills will help you to assess the casualty's condition, and explain what you are doing and why.

Some rules for effective communication:

- Be calm and direct
- Be respectful
- Do not use medical terms
- Call the casualty by name
- Do not diagnose the casualty's condition
- Always be honest, reassuring, and choose your words carefully

As a first aider, the first thing you do when you arrive at an emergency scene is take charge of the situation. You stay in charge until you hand control of the scene over to more qualified people. While in charge, many other people may offer to help.

When handing the scene over to someone other than the casualty, describe the complete history of the incident and pass along any notes you have taken. Be sure to include:

- your name
- the time you arrived
- the history of the illness or injury, including signs and symptoms observed
- what first aid has been given
- any changes in the casualty's condition since you took charge

1

Principles of communication

Though each situation is different, the following general guidelines help improve communication.

Focus

Maintain your attention on the casualty. Position yourself at eye level and maintain eye contact.

Terminology

Refrain from using medical terminology when communicating with the casualty or bystanders. Explanations and answers must be clear, concise and easily understood.

Body Language

Refrain from using body language that could be perceived as threatening or aggressive.

Professionalism

Always maintain your professionalism. Explain everything you are doing and why. If what you are doing may be painful, let the casualty know.

Injuries and illness

Injuries

When something from outside the body damages tissues, the damaged area is called an injury. How serious an injury is depends on:

- **what tissues are injured**—an injury to a vital organ, or tissues of a vital system, like the nervous system, is serious

- **how bad the injury is**—for instance, a bone broken in half may not be as serious as the same bone shattered into many pieces

- **how much tissue is injured**—a burned hand may be more serious than a burned finger

Injuries and energy

Injuries result from too much energy being applied to the body. For instance:

- a thermal burn is caused by too much heat energy
- an acid burn is caused by too much chemical energy
- snow-blindness is caused by too much light energy
- a broken bone is caused by too much mechanical energy
- a stopped heart from an electric shock is caused by too much electrical energy

The body can take a certain amount of energy without being injured. But too much of any sort of energy will cause injury. Three factors determine whether an injury will occur. They are:

- how intense the energy was
- how long the energy was applied to the body
- what part of the body the energy was applied to

Most injuries are caused either by something hitting the body or the body hitting something—this is mechanical energy. When something moves, it has mechanical energy. How much mechanical energy something has depends on how fast it is moving and how much it weighs.

Illness

We often think of first aid in the context of injuries only. But when someone becomes very sick, the result can be a medical emergency in which first aid can save a life.

Some illnesses, like heart attacks or strokes come on very fast. Other illnesses progress more slowly and it can be hard to decide exactly when you have a medical problem that calls for a doctor's attention.

1

Get medical help when any of the following is present:

- sudden severe pain in any part of the body
- sudden changes in vision, headache or dizziness
- severe or persistent diarrhea or vomiting
- sudden weakness or slurred/jumbled speech
- persistent high temperature
- changes in level of consciousness
- skin rash of unknown origin
- repeated fainting
- obvious depression, suicide threats or attempts
- whenever you are very worried about yourself or someone in your care

If the casualty is an infant, the following are also reasons to get medical help (in addition to the reasons above):

- the baby has had a seizure
- the baby is blue or very pale
- you think the baby is having trouble breathing
- the baby cries a lot, or won't stop crying

Stress management in emergency situations

First aiders may experience a certain level of stress as a result of the assistance they provide. Stress is the body's normal reaction to physical and psychological events. It can be seen in certain attitudes and behaviors in both casualties and first aiders. It is a biological response and may be reflected in:

- an increase in heart rate
- an increase in blood pressure
- an increase in blood sugar
- dilation of the bronchi and pupils

Possible reactions of casualties

Casualties may react to stressors in different ways and first aiders must observe and adjust to such reactions which can include:

- **denial**—the casualty may deny the seriousness of the situation and refuse assistance

- **resignation**—the casualty may be resigned to dying even if their life does not seem to be in danger, and doesn't want to make any effort to do what is needed

- **aggressiveness**—the casualty may be hostile

- **assertiveness**—the casualty is positive, cooperative, and may even want to take charge of their own care including directing the first aiders

Stress management

Managing stress in an emergency situation can make a significant difference in the quality of first aid provided. Appropriate mental preparation and regular first aid skill practice can help first aiders react effectively when faced with an emergency situation. The negative impact of stress can be reduced by understanding it and taking measures to try and overcome it. After serious incidents, it is important for first aiders to process their emotions.

When faced with a highly stressful situation some first aiders may experience prolonged effects of stress and they should seek medical assistance.

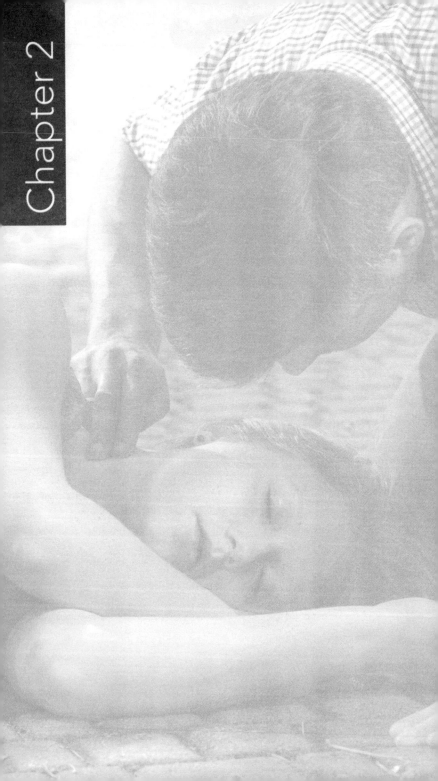

Emergency Scene Management

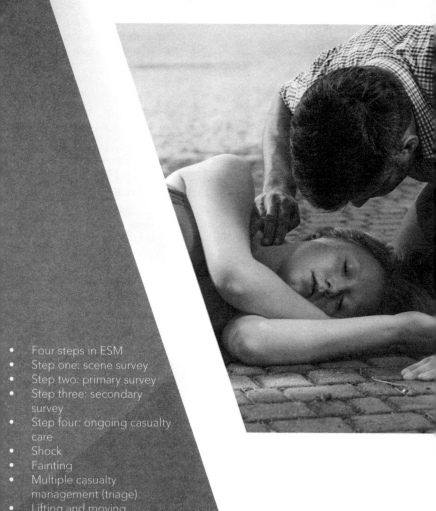

- Four steps in ESM
- Step one: scene survey
- Step two: primary survey
- Step three: secondary survey
- Step four: ongoing casualty care
- Shock
- Fainting
- Multiple casualty management (triage)
- Lifting and moving

Chapter 2 Emergency scene management

Emergency scenes generally begin with confusion as people realize there is an emergency unfolding in front of them. No one knows what to do first, who should be in charge, or how they can help. In this situation, the first aider needs to follow a sequence of actions that ensures safe and appropriate first aid is given and everyone's safety is protected. First aiders use emergency scene management (ESM) to do this. Emergency scene management is the sequence of actions you should follow to ensure safe and appropriate first aid is given.

Four steps in ESM:

1. **scene survey**—during the scene survey you take control of the scene, find out what happened and make sure the area is safe before assessing the casualty

2. **primary survey**—assess each casualty for life-threatening injuries and illnesses, and give life-saving first aid

3. **secondary survey**—the secondary survey is a step-by-step way of gathering information to form a complete picture of the casualty's overall condition

4. **ongoing casualty care**—during ongoing casualty care you continue to monitor the casualty's condition until medical help takes over

These steps are generally done in the order above. The initial scene survey, primary survey and the start of life-saving first aid usually happens within one or two minutes. The secondary survey is not always necessary.

Step one: scene survey

- Take charge of the situation
- Call out for help to attract bystanders
- Assess hazards and make the area safe
- Find out the history of the emergency, how many casualties there are and the mechanism(s) of injury
- Identify yourself as a first aider and offer to help, get consent
- Assess responsiveness

2

Send or go for medical help as soon as you identify a serious problem and then begin the primary survey. If you have a mobile phone, you can dial 9-1-1 or your local emergency number, and put the device on speaker phone, if possible. This allows the first aider to remain with the casualty.

Step two: primary survey

Check for life-threatening conditions, the ABCs:

A = Airway

B = Breathing

C = Circulation

The sequential steps of the primary survey should be performed with the casualty in the position found unless it is impossible to do so.

The primary survey should begin immediately after the scene survey.

2

1. Check the airway

If the casualty is conscious, ask "what happened?" How well the casualty responds will help you determine if the airway is clear. Use a head-tilt-chin-lift to open the airway of an unresponsive casualty.

If you suspect a head or spinal injury and have been trained, use a jaw-thrust without head-tilt.

2. Check for breathing

If the casualty is conscious, check by asking how their breathing is.

If the casualty is unconscious, check for breathing for at least five seconds, and no more than 10 seconds. If breathing is effective, move on to check circulation. If breathing is absent or ineffective (gasping and irregular, agonal), begin CPR.

3. Check circulation

- Control obvious, severe bleeding
- Check for shock by checking skin condition and temperature
- Check with a rapid body survey for hidden, severe, external bleeding and signs of internal bleeding

Rapid body survey

The rapid body survey is a quick assessment of the casualty's body which is performed during the primary survey. By running your hands over the casualty's entire body from head to toe (and under heavy outwear), you are able to feel for severe bleeding, internal bleeding and any obvious fractures.

When performing the rapid body survey:

- Wear gloves when possible, and check gloves for blood every few seconds

- Be careful not to cause any further injuries while performing the survey

2

- Look at the casualty's face to notice any responses to the rapid body survey

Provide first aid for life-threatening injuries or conditions.

- Maintain an open airway with a head-tilt chin-lift or by placing the unresponsive breathing casualty into the recovery position

- Provide CPR if the unresponsive casualty is not breathing or not breathing normally (gasping)

- Control severe bleeding

- Provide support for obvious fractures

- Give first aid for shock by providing first aid for life-threatening injuries and maintaining the casualty's body temperature

Evaluate the situation and decide whether to do a secondary survey

Do a secondary survey if:

- the casualty has more than one injury

- medical help will be delayed more than 20 minutes

- medical help is not coming to the scene and you have to transport the casualty

If you do not do a secondary survey, steady and support any injuries found and give ongoing casualty care until medical help arrives.

How to turn a casualty face up

2

You should give first aid in the position in which the casualty is found as much as possible. But sometimes you have to turn a casualty over to assess for life-threatening injuries or to give life-saving first aid.

1   Extend the arm closest to you over the head.

2   Tuck the far arm against the casualty's side.

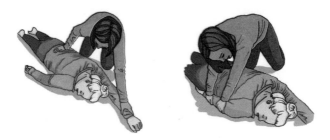

3   Cross the far foot over the near foot.

4   Support the head and neck. Firmly grip the clothing at the waist. Roll the casualty over.

5   Position the casualty for giving first aid.

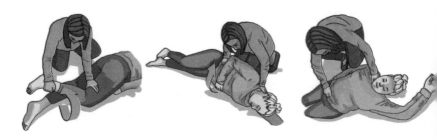

ESM when a head or spinal injury is suspected

If you suspect a head or spinal injury, protect the head and neck from any movement. Head or neck movement could result in life-long disability or death. Adjust your first aid to this situation as shown below.

2

1   As soon as you see there might be a head or spinal injury, tell the casualty not to move.

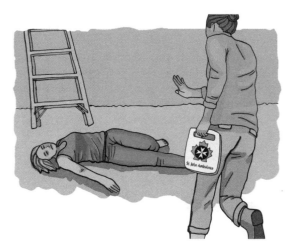

2   Once you have consent to help the casualty, steady and support the head and neck. Keep elbows firmly supported on thighs or ground. Then, assess responsiveness.

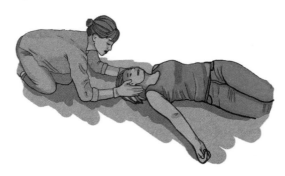

2

3   If there is a bystander to help, show them how to support the head and neck so you can continue your assessment.

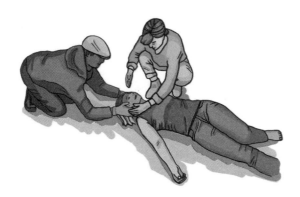

4   Continue your assessment.

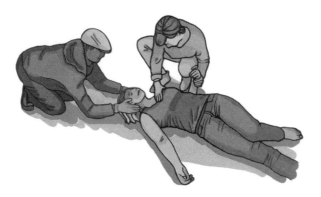

2

5   If a second bystander is available, show them how to steady and support the feet to prevent movement.

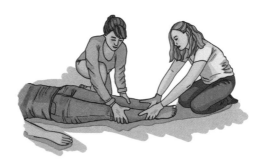

6   Keep the head and neck supported (and the feet if possible) while giving further first aid until handover to medical help.

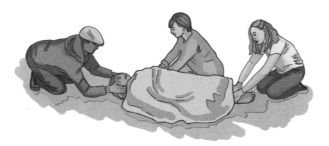

When **moving a casualty** with a suspected head or spinal injury, move them as a unit as much as possible. This means rolling the head, trunk and legs together, or lifting the whole body at the same time. Do what you can to prevent movement.

Turning a casualty face up when a head or spinal injury is suspected

2

You should give first aid in the position in which the casualty is found as much as possible. But sometimes you have to turn a casualty over to assess for life-threatening injuries or give life-saving first aid.

When you suspect a head or spinal injury, turn the casualty as a unit so the head and spine stay in the same relative position.

1   The first aider at the head supports the head—placing the right hand along the right side of the casualty's head and the left hand along the left side.

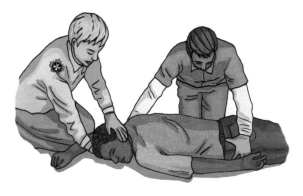

2   The other first aider extends the casualty's near arm over their head and gets a good grip on the casualty at the shoulder and waist.

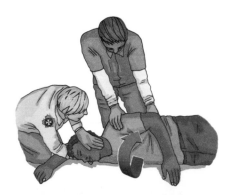

At the same time, the two first aiders roll the casualty towards the second first aider.

3   If extra help is available, have the third first aider support the legs to prevent twisting of the neck and spine. With a fourth, put one first aider at the shoulders and another at the waist.

2

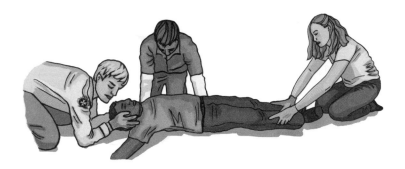

Step three: secondary survey

A **secondary survey** follows the primary survey and any life-saving first aid. It is a step-by-step way of gathering information to form a complete picture of the casualty. In the secondary survey, the first aider is looking for injuries or illnesses that may not have been revealed in the primary survey. You should complete a secondary survey if:

- the casualty has more than one injury
- medical help will be delayed for 20 minutes or more
- you will transport the casualty to medical help

The secondary survey has four steps:

1. History
2. Vital signs
3. Head-to-toe exam
4. First aid for any injury or illness found

History

A **SAMPLE** history is used to gather a brief medical history of the casualty. This information may be useful for health care professionals who will continue to assist the casualty. If the casualty is unable to respond, some of the SAMPLE history could be answered by a close family member.

S = **symptoms** – what the casualty is feeling (such as pain, nausea, weakness, etc.)

A = **allergies** – any allergies, specifically allergies to medications

M = **medications** – any medications or supplements they normally take, have taken in the past 24 hours, or any doses they may have missed

P = **past or present medical history** – any medical history, especially if it is related to what they are experiencing now. Ask if they have medical alert information

L = **last meal** – last meal they ate and when, anything else taken by mouth

E = **events leading to the incident** – what was happening before the injury/illness? How did the injury occur?

2

Vital signs

There are four vital signs to check on the casualty

1. Level of consciousness (LOC)
2. Breathing
3. Pulse
4. Skin condition and temperature

Level of consciousness (LOC)

A common method of obtaining a casualty's LOC is using the acronym **AVPU**. When using AVPU to indicate LOC, it is a scale which ranges from good (A), to not as good (V), to bad (P), to worse (U)

A = **Alert** – An alert casualty will have their eyes open and will be able to answer simple questions. An alert casualty is oriented to person, place and time.

V = **Verbal** – The casualty will respond when spoken to, but may not be able to effectively communicate. They may not be oriented to person, place or time.

P = **Pain** – This casualty will only respond when a painful stimuli is delivered, such as pinching them or rubbing your knuckles on their sternum. They may move or make noise, but they will not communicate.

U = **Unresponsive** – the unresponsive casualty will not respond to any stimulus.

Please note that an alternative to quickly estimate a casualty's LOC is to evaluate their eye, verbal and motor skills. If their eyes are open, they can clearly speak, and obey a command such as "squeeze my fingers," they are alert.

Breathing

To assess the breathing rate, watch the casualty closely for a total of 30 seconds. It is OK to place your hand on their upper abdomen to feel the rise and fall. Check the quality of the breathing. Carefully count each breath over the 30 seconds and multiply that number by two for breaths per minute.

Normal breathing rates			
Age	Too slow	Normal	Too fast
Infant	Below 25	30-50	Above 60
Child	Below 15	20-30	Above 40
Adult	Below 10	10-20	Above 30

Pulse

The pulse rate is the number of beats your heart takes in one minute, and it is an essential skill for assessing all casualties. The most common places to assess a pulse is at the wrist or neck, and for infants, the inside of the upper arm.

To assess the pulse, use two fingers and gently place them on either the inside of the wrist (just below the hand on the thumb side), or on the side of the neck (carotid artery), or for infants, the inside of

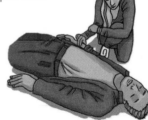

the upper arm, on the brachial artery. Press just gently enough to feel the pulse. You may have to feel around the area until you find it. Once you have found the pulse, count the number of beats over 30 seconds and multiply that number by two.

Normal pulse rates	
Age	Normal pulse range
Infant	120-150
Child	80-150
Adult	60-100

Skin condition and temperature

When assessing the skin we look for the temperature (warm or cold), the colour (normal skin tones or pale) and whether the skin is dry or wet. Use the back of your gloved hand to feel the casualty's forehead and cheeks. If their skin normal, they will have normal skin

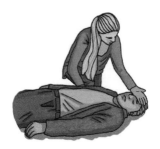

colour, and their skin will be warm and dry. If the skin is pale, cold and wet (sweaty), this could be an indication of shock.

Head-to-toe exam

The head-to-toe exam is a complete and detailed check of the casualty for any injuries that may have been missed during the rapid body survey. **Do not examine for unlikely injuries.** You may need to expose an area to check for injuries, but always respect the casualty's modesty and ensure you protect them from the cold. Only expose what you absolutely have to.

- Ask the casualty if they feel any pain before you start. Note any responses.

- Speak to the casualty throughout the process. Explain what you are checking for as you proceed.

- Always watch the casualty's face for any facial expressions that may indicate pain.

- Do not stop the exam. If you find an injury, note it and continue.

- Do not step over the casualty. If you need to, walk around them.

- During a detailed exam, you are looking for all bumps, bruises, scrapes, or anything that is not normal.

- If the casualty is unconscious, look for medic alert devices during your survey, such as a tag, bracelet, necklace, watch, or other idicator.

Look, then feel

Start at the head:

- Check the skull for anything abnormal
- Check the ears for fluid
- Check the eyes, are the pupils the same size?
- Check the nose for drainage
- Check the mouth, are the teeth intact? Are the lips blue or pale?

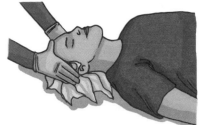

Check the neck:

- Are the neck veins bulging?
- Is there a medical alert necklace?
- Check the collarbones
- Check the shoulders on both sides

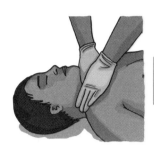

Check the arms:

- Check each arm completely
- Check the fingernails for circulation by squeezing and watching the blood return
- Ask the casualty to squeeze two of your fingers in both hands at the same time. Do they have an adequate strength and is the strength equal?

Check the chest and under:

- Does it hurt the casualty to breathe?
- Does the chest rise and fall with breaths as it should?
- Reach around the back as far as you can

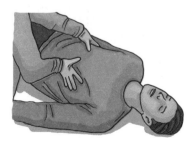

2

Check the abdomen and under:

- With flat hands, check the abdomen carefully
- Do not push into the abdomen. Gently feel for pain, tenderness, or rigidity
- Place a flat hand on their abdomen and ask the casualty to push against it. Does this cause pain?
- Reach around the back as far as you can

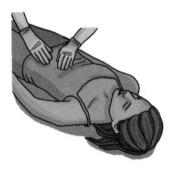

Check the pelvis:

- Place your hands on top of the pelvic bones and very gently squeeze for stability

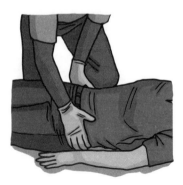

Check the legs, ankles, and feet:

- Check each leg completely one at a time
- Is one leg shorter than the other?
- Carefully check the stability of the kneecap and under the knee
- Squeeze or pinch a foot. Ask the casualty what you just did to see if they answer correctly.
- Place both hands on both feet. Ask the casualty to push and then pull against you. Feel for equal strength. Ask the casualty to wiggle their toes and watch for the response.
- Check circulation

2

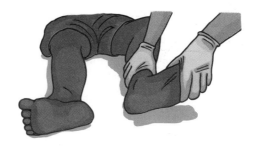

Check the back:

- Check the back when the casualty is rolled onto a stretcher or you need to move them for a specific reason.
- Be careful to not aggravate any injuries if moving the casualty.

First aid for injuries found

When you have completed your exam, give appropriate first aid for any injuries or illnesses found. If the casualty has more than one injury, give first aid to the more serious injuries first.

Document

Upon completion of the secondary survey, document your findings as accurately as possible. This information may be valuable to medical professionals who will continue to assist the casualty.

Step four: ongoing casualty care

Once first aid for injuries and illnesses that are not life threatening has been given:

- the first aider will hand over control of the scene to the casualty, or someone else, and end there involvement in the emergency
- the first aider will stay in control of the scene and wait for medical help to take over, or
- the first aider will stay in control of the scene and transport the casualty to medical help

The first aid must maintain the casualty in the best possible condition until handover to medical help by:

- Giving first aid for shock
- Monitoring the casualty's condition
- Recording the events of the situation
- Reporting on what happened to whoever takes over

Instruct a bystander to maintain manual support of the head and neck (if head/spinal injuries are suspected). Continue to steady and support manually, if needed.

How to put a casualty into the recovery position

This position protects the casualty and also reduces bending and twisting of the spine. This position protects the airway if you must leave the casualty.

2

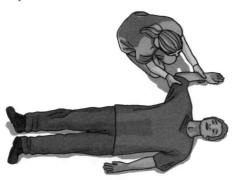

1   Position the arm closest to you at 90 degrees in front of the casualty, keeping it out of the way when rolling them.

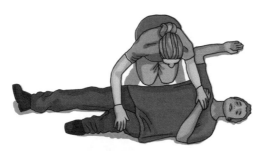

2   Position the arm furthest from you on the casualty's chest. Bend the far knee.

2

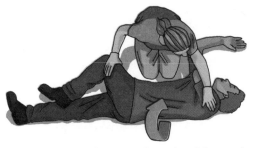

3   Reach behind the casualty's shoulder and roll casualty towards you by pulling on the far knee.

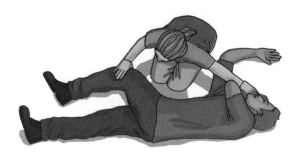

4   Adjust the position of the arms and leg so the casualty is in a stable position. Place the far arm at 90 degrees to the casualty with the palm down.

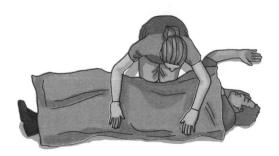

5   Give ongoing care.

After the handover

In first aid, we prepare ourselves to care for an injured or ill person. We don't often think about what happens after the casualty has left our care. Immediately following the handover of the casualty you may have a number of practical details to attend to. These details can include cleaning up after the emergency, correcting any unsafe conditions that caused the injury, or making a report on the incident and your involvement.

Once these practical matters are out of the way, we expect things to "return to normal." However, you will likely find yourself thinking about the situation and the details of what happened while you were involved. Following a stressful event, many people review the details and try to evaluate what they did and how they could have done it better.

This reviewing of the events is completely normal and you can expect it to happen. But if thoughts of the incident continue for many weeks, or if they affect your day-to-day life, you may be experiencing the negative effects of critical incident stress (CIS).

Critical incident stress is a common reaction to a stressful emergency situation. The effects of CIS can interfere with your daily life—your job, your relationships, your peace of mind. If this happens to you, you need to do something about it, and help is readily available. Start by talking to your family doctor or a doctor at a walk-in clinic. A doctor will understand what you are going through and will suggest a course of action.

The effects of critical incident stress can appear many weeks, months or years after the event.

Shock

Shock is a circulation problem where the body's tissues don't get enough oxygenated blood.

2

Shock is a danger because any physical injury or illness can be accompanied by shock, and it can quickly progress into a life-threatening condition. Pain, anxiety and fear do not cause shock, but they can make it worse, or make it progress faster. This is why reassuring a casualty and making them comfortable is important.

Medical shock should not be confused with electrical shock or being shocked and surprised. Medical shock is life-threatening, as the brain and other organs cannot function properly.

The following information provides some causes of shock. Severe shock can also result from medical emergencies such as diabetes, epilepsy, infection, poisoning or a drug overdose.

Common causes of severe shock	
Cause of shock	How it causes a circulation problem
severe bleeding - internal or external (includes major fractures)	not enough blood to fill blood vessels
severe burns	loss of blood plasma (fluid) into tissues—not enough blood to fill blood vessels
crush injuries	loss of blood and blood plasma into tissues—not enough blood to fill blood vessels
heart attack	heart is not strong enough to pump blood effectively
spinal cord or nerve injuries	brain can't control the size of the blood vessels—the blood can't get to the tissues properly
severe allergic reactions	many things can be affected—breathing, heart function, etc.

Signs and symptoms of shock

Signs	Symptoms
• pale skin at first, turns blue-grey*	• restless
• blue-purple lips, tongue, earlobes, fingernails	• anxious
• cold and clammy skin	• disoriented
• breathing shallow and irregular, fast or gasping for air	• confused
• changes in level of consciousness	• afraid
• weak, rapid pulse—radial pulse may be absent	• dizzy
	• thristy

*For casualties with dark skin colour, colour changes may be observed in the following areas of the body: lips, gums and tongue, nail beds and palms, earlobes, membrane of the inner eyelid.

2

First aid for shock

The following actions will minimize shock:

1. Give first aid for the injury or illness that caused the shock
2. Reassure the casualty often
3. Minimize pain by handling the casualty gently
4. Loosen tight clothing at the neck, chest and waist
5. Keep the casualty warm, but do not overheat — use jackets, coats or blankets if you have them
6. Moisten the lips if the casualty complains of thirst. Don't give anything to eat or drink. If medical help is delayed many hours, give small amounts of water or clear fluids to drink — make a note of what was given and when
7. Place the casualty in the best position for their condition Continue ongoing casualty care until handover

The above first aid for shock may prevent shock from getting worse. Whenever possible, add these steps to any first aid you give.

Positioning a casualty in shock

Putting the casualty in the right position can slow the progress of shock and make the casualty more comfortable.

The position you use depends on the casualty's condition. The casualty should be as comfortable as possible in the position you use.

No suspected head/spinal injury; fully conscious

Place the casualty on their back, if injuries permit. Once the casualty is positioned, cover them to preserve body heat, but do not overheat.

No suspected head/spinal injury; less than fully conscious

Place the casualty in the recovery position. When there is decreased level of consciousness, airway and breathing are the priority—the recovery position ensures an open airway.

Conscious with a breathing emergency and/or chest pain

If a conscious casualty is experiencing chest pain or is having difficulty breathing, have them sit in a semi-sitting position, or any position that makes breathing easier for them.

Suspected head/spinal injury

If you suspect a head or spinal injury, steady and support the casualty in the position found. This protects the head and spine from further injury. Monitor the ABCs closely.

As injuries permit

A casualty's injuries may not permit you to put them into the best position. Continue to support the head and neck and, if needed, use a head-tilt chin-lift to maintain the open airway. Always think of the casualty's comfort when choosing a position.

Fainting

Fainting is a temporary loss of consciousness caused by a shortage of oxygenated blood to the brain. Common causes of fainting include:

- Fear or anxiety
- Lack of fresh air
- Severe pain, injury or illness
- The sight of blood
- An underlying medical problem
- Fatigue or hunger
- Long periods of standing or sitting
- Overheating

A person who has fainted is unconscious. Place them in recovery position to protect the airway and prevent possible choking. Place the casualt in a comfortable position as they regain consciousness.

First aid for fainting

- Ensure a supply of fresh air and loosen tight clothing at the neck, chest and waist.

- Make the casualty comfortable as consciousness returns and keep them lying down for 10 to 15 minutes. Continue to monitor breathing and consciousness.

Do not assume a person has "just fainted," unless there is a quick recovery. If the recovery is not quick or complete, stay with the casualty until medical help takes over.

If you have to leave to get medical help or you have to give first aid to other casualties, turn the casualty into the recovery position being as careful as you can if there are any injuries.

Feeling faint or "impending faint"

Sometimes when a person is about to faint, there are warning signs. The person:

- is pale

- is sweating

- feels sick, nauseous, dizzy or unsteady

First aid for an impending faint

1. Place the casualty on their back.

2. Ensure a supply of fresh air—open windows or doors.

3. Loosen tight clothing at the neck, chest and waist.

4. Stay with the casualty until they has fully recovered.

Decreased level of consciousness (LOC)

Consciousness refers to the level of awareness one has of themselves and their surroundings. There are different levels of consciousness ranging from completely conscious to completely unconscious. Many injuries/illnesses can cause changes in a casualty's level of consciousness, including:

- a breathing emergency
- a heart attack
- a head injury
- poisoning
- shock
- alcohol or drug abuse
- medical condition (epilepsy, diabetes, etc.)

Semi-consciousness and unconsciousness are breathing emergencies for casualties lying on their back, because the tongue may fall to the back of the throat and block the airway. Saliva and other fluids can also pool at the back of the throat and choke the person.

A progressive loss of consciousness means the casualty's condition is getting worse. Always monitor a casualty's level of consciousness and note any changes. A first aider can use the acronym AVPU (alert, verbal, pain, unresponsive) to assess and describe levels of consciousness.

Decreased consciousness is always an urgent situation. The person can quickly become unconscious, and this is a breathing emergency. When you recognize decreased consciousness, get medical help as quickly as possible.

First aid for unconsciousness

1. Start ESM. Perform a scene survey. Call or send for medical help as soon as unresponsiveness is determined.

2. Do a primary survey.

3. Do a secondary survey if necessary.

4. Turn the casualty into the recovery position, if injuries permit. Give ongoing care.

If injuries make it necessary for the casualty to be face up, monitor breathing continuously. If necessary, hold the airway open. Always ensure an open airway.

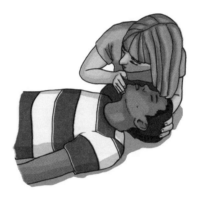

5. Loosen tight clothing at the neck, chest and waist, and continue ongoing casualty care until handover. Record any changes in level of consciousness and when they happen.

A decreased consciousness also requires urgent medical help.

Multiple casualty management (triage)

The process of making decisions at an emergency scene where multiple people are injured is called **triage**. In triage, first aiders quickly examine all casualties and place them in order of greatest need for first aid and for transportation. The idea is to do the most good for the greatest number of casualties.

2

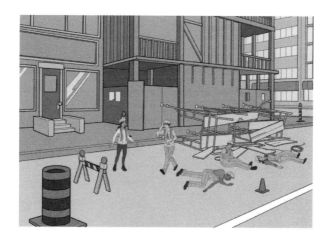

Casualties are categorized into three levels of priority:

- **highest priority**—casualties who need immediate first aid and transportation to medical help

- **medium priority**—casualties who probably can wait one hour for medical help without risk to their lives

- **lowest priority**—casualties who can wait and receive first aid and transportation last, or casualties who are obviously dead

Note: in the event of a lightning strike, where more than one person is injured, the principles of multiple casualty management are reversed. Give first aid to unresponsive non-breathing casualties since the casualties that are still breathing are recovering.

The first aid priorities for injuries

Priority	Condition	Causes
High priority Airway	foreign body blocking airway	choking on food
	tongue or fluids blocking airway	unconscious, lying on back
	swollen airway	allergic reaction, airway infection
High priority Breathing	injured chest and/or lungs	chest injury, broken ribs
	brain not controlling breathing properly	poisoning, drug overdose, stroke, electric shock
	not enough oxygen reaching blood	not enough oxygen in air, carbon monoxide poisoning
High priority Circulation	severe bleeding	external bleeding or internal bleeding
	severe shock	bleeding, serious illness, poisoning
Medium priority Injuries that may affect ABCs or have potential for life-long disability	fractures that could affect breathing	broken ribs, shoulder blade
	fractures—open, severe or multiple bones	broken upper leg, pelvis, crushed arm
	head/spinal injuries	fall from a six-foot ladder
	critical burns	critical burns to the hands
Low priority Minor injuries or obviously dead	minor fractures	broken lower leg, lower arm, hand, finger, etc.
	minor bleeding	bleeding not spurting or free-flowing
	non-critical burns	moderate degree burns to the forearms
	behavioural problems	grief or panic
	obviously dead	obvious massive injuries, no pulse or other signs of circulation

2

Triage sequence of actions

1. Begin ESM
   - Determine how many casualties there are in the scene survey.
2. Start with the nearest casualty, and move outward
   - Do a primary survey
   - Give first aid for life-threatening injuries
   - If the person is obviously dead, go to the next nearest casualty
3. Repeat step 2 for each casualty
   - Always move to the next nearest casualty
4. Categorize
   - Decide which casualties have the highest priority, second priority, and lowest priority.
5. Arrange transportation
   - Arrange for the highest priority casualties to be transported to medical help as soon as possible
6. Perform secondary survey
   - Begin with the highest priority. Give appropriate first aid, and move on
7. Give ongoing care for each casualty until transported

In a multiple casualty situation, constantly assess the casualties and the situation and make changes to priorities.

Lifting and moving

Always try to give necessary first aid where the casualty is found, then wait for the paramedics to move the person. However, there are times when this is not possible.

You may have to move a casualty when:

- there are life-threatening hazards to yourself or the casualty e.g. danger from fire, explosion, gas or water

- essential first aid for wounds or other conditions cannot be given in the casualty's present position or location

- the casualty must be transported to a medical facility

If life-threatening hazards make it necessary to move a casualty right away, you may need to use a rescue carry.

In urgent and dangerous situations where casualties are moved with less than ideal support for injuries, the casualty's injuries may be made worse by improper movement and handling. The chance of further injury can be reduced with proper rescue carry techniques.

Always move the casualty the shortest possible distance to safety and to provide essential first aid. Use bystanders to help you and support any injuries the best you can during the move. Keep the risks to the casualty, yourself and others to a minimum.

Lifting techniques and proper body mechanics

Moving any casualty from an emergency scene poses dangers to the rescuer as well as the casualty. If the casualty must be moved, select the method that will pose the least risk to the casualty and to you. You can be of little help to a casualty if you injure yourself in the rescue.

2

Using incorrect body mechanics in lifting or moving a casualty may leave the rescuer suffering muscle strains. Use the following lifting guidelines:

1   Stand close to the object to be lifted.

2   Bend your knees, not your waist.

3   Tilt the object so that you can put one hand under the edge or corner closest to you.

4   Place your other hand under the opposite side or corner, getting a good grip on the object.

5   Use your leg muscles to lift, and keep your back straight.

6   When turning, turn your feet first; don't twist your body.

When lowering the object, reverse the procedure.

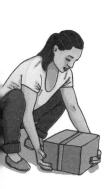
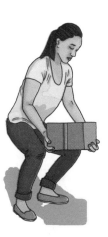
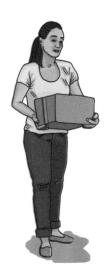

Rescue carries

A rescue carry is an emergency method of moving a casualty over a short distance to safety, shelter or to transportation. Select the type of carry based on the circumstances.

- the size and weight of the casualty relative to the rescuer
- the number of rescuers available to assist
- the type of injury
- the distance to move the casualty

Whenever possible, ask one or more bystanders to help you. When help is available:

- remain with the casualty
- give instructions to the bystanders about what to do and what safety precautions to take
- fully coordinate the rescue activities

Drag carry

This carry is used by the single rescuer to drag a casualty who is either lying on their back or in a sitting position. The drag carry provides maximum protection to the head and neck, and therefore should be used when you are moving a casualty with this type of injury.

If time permits, tie the casualty's wrists together across their chest before dragging.

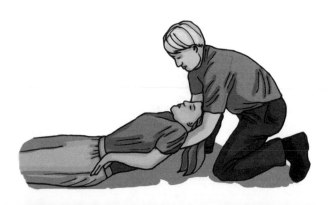

1   Stand at the casualty's head facing their feet.

2   Crouch down and ease your hands under the casualty's shoulders. Grasp the clothing on each side. Support the casualty's head between your forearms to stop movement.

3   Drag the casualty backward only as far as necessary for their safety.

As an alternate method, the first aider can use a blanket to support and drag the casualty.

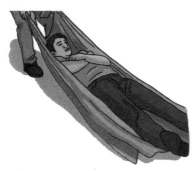

Because of the risk of aggravating any injuries, only use drag carries in the most extreme cases when there is an immediate threat to life.

Human crutch

If a leg or foot is injured, help the casualty to walk on their good leg while you give support to the injured side.

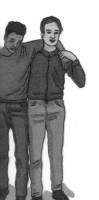

1   Take the weight of the casualty's injured side on your shoulders by placing the casualty's arm (on the injured side) around your neck and grasping the wrist firmly.

2   Reach around the casualty's back with your free hand, and grasp the clothing at the waist.

3   Tell the casualty to step off with you, each using the inside foot. This lets you, the rescuer; take the casualty's weight on the injured side.

Chair carry

The chair carry enables two rescuers to carry a conscious or unconscious casualty through narrow passages and up and down stairs. Do not use this carry for casualties with suspected neck or back injuries. Specially designed rescue chairs are available and should be used for this type of carry.

If the casualty is unconscious or helpless:

1   Place an unconscious casualty on a chair by sliding the back of the chair under their legs and buttocks, and along the lower back.

2   Strap their upper body and arms to the back of the chair.

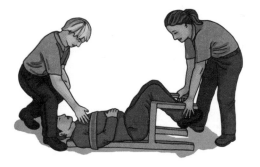

3   Two rescuers carry the chair, one at the front and one at the back. The rescuer at the back crouches and grasps the back of the chair, while the rescuer at the front crouches between the casualty's knees and grasps the front chair legs near the floor.

4   The rescuers walk out-of-step.

Going down stairs

• The casualty faces forward

• The front rescuer faces the casualty

• A third person should act as a guide and support the front rescuer in case they lose their footing

Extremity carry

Use the extremity carry when you don't have a chair and do not
suspect fractures of the trunk, head, or spine.

1 One rescuer passes their hands under
the casualty's armpits, and grasps the
casualty's wrists, crossing them over their
chest.

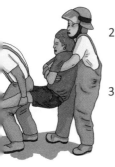

2 The second rescuer crouches with their
back between the casualty's knees and
grasps each leg just above the knee.

3 The rescuers step off on opposite feet—
walking out-of-step is smoother for the
casualty.

Blanket lift with four bearers

1 Roll the blanket or rug lengthwise for half its width.
Position bearers at the head and feet to keep the head,
neck and body in line. Place the rolled edge along the
casualty's injured side.

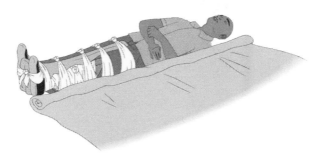

2 Kneel at the casualty's shoulder and position another
bearer at the waist to help logroll the casualty onto
the uninjured side. Turn the casualty as a unit so the
casualty's body is not twisted.

3 Roll the casualty back over the blanket roll to lay face
up on the blanket. Unroll the blanket and then roll the

2

edges of the blanket to each side of the casualty. Get ready to lift the casualty—have the bearers grip the rolls at the head and shoulders, and at the hip and legs.

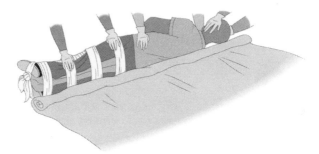

4   Keep the blanket tight as the casualty is lifted and placed on the stretcher.

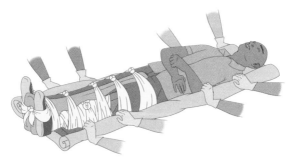

Before using a blanket, test it to ensure that it will carry the casualty's weight. Do not use this lift if neck or back injuries are suspected.

Stretchers

There may be times when medical help cannot be contacted, or for other reasons, cannot come to the scene. When this happens, transport the casualty to medical help. If the casualty can't walk, or if the injury or illness allows only the gentlest movement, a stretcher should be used.

Commercial stretchers

The most common of the commercial stretchers is the rigid-pole, canvas stretcher. It has hinged bracing bars at right angles between the rigid poles at either end that must be locked in the extended position before the stretcher is used.

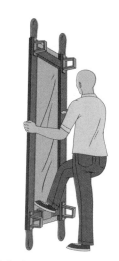

Improvised stretchers

If a commercially prepared stretcher is not available, you can improvise one by using two rigid poles and a blanket, clothing or grain sacks. Do not use non-rigid stretchers for casualties with suspected head or spinal injuries.

Principles for stretcher use

Complete all essential first aid and immobilization before moving the casualty onto a stretcher.

- Bring the blanketed and padded stretcher to the casualty, rather than moving the casualty to the stretcher.

- As the first aider in charge, take the position that permits you to watch and control the most sensitive area of the body, usually at the head and shoulders, or the injured part.

- Tell the bearers what each is expected to do. If the move is difficult, and time permits, it's a good idea to practice with a simulated casualty. This reduces risks and reassures the conscious casualty.

- Test an improvised stretcher with someone equal to or heavier than the casualty to ensure that it will hold.

- Check the clearance of an improvised stretcher to ensure that it will pass through hallways, doors and stairways without harm to the casualty. Use clear commands to ensure smooth, coordinated movements.

Improvised blanket stretcher

1. Place the blanket flat on the ground and place a pole one-third of the way from one end. Fold the one-third length of blanket over the pole.

2. Place the second pole parallel to the first so that it is on the doubled part of the blanket, about 15 cm (6 inches) from the doubled edge.

3. Fold the remaining blanket over the two poles. The casualty's weight on the blanket holds the folds in place.

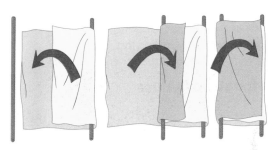

Improvised jacket stretcher

A non-rigid stretcher can also be improvised from two jackets and two or four poles.

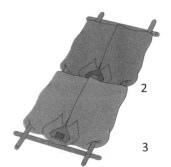

1. Button and zipper the jackets closed and pull the sleeves inside out so that the sleeves are inside. Lay the jackets on the ground so that the top edge of one jacket meets the bottom edge of the other.

2. Pass the poles through the sleeves of the two jackets on either side to complete the stretcher.

3. If the casualty is tall, prepare another jacket as before and add it to the stretcher with the head of the jacket towards the middle.

Four-bearer method—no blanket

1   All bearers kneel on their left knees, three on one side of the casualty and one on the other, as shown below. Bearer 4 helps in lifting and lowering the casualty, and also places the stretcher under the casualty.

2   Bearer 4 joins hands with bearers 1 and 2. When assured that each bearer has a firm hold on the casualty, bearer 1 directs the others to "Get ready to lift" and then gives the command "Lift." Lift the casualty smoothly to the height of the raised knees.

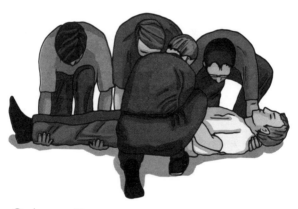

3   On bearer 1's command "Rest," the casualty is gently laid on the raised knees of bearers 1, 2 and 3.

4   Bearer 1 tells bearer 4 to position the stretcher. Bearer 4 then resumes their position supporting the casualty by linking their hands with one from each of bearers 1 and 2.

5   Position the stretcher.

6   When everyone is in position, bearer 1 instructs the team to, "Get ready to lower" and then, "lower." The team lowers the casualty gently onto the stretcher. Secure the casualty to the stretcher.

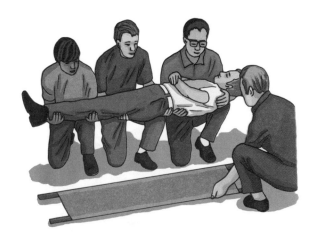

Three-bearer method, no blanket

The three-bearer method is essentially the same as the four-bearer method, except the first aider and one bearer share the weight on one side of the casualty. The third bearer links hands with the first aider from the opposite side to take up the weight of the trunk. The casualty is lifted and rested on the bearers' knees while the stretcher is positioned and bearer 3 links hands again with the first aider to help lower the casualty to the stretcher.

Carrying a stretcher

A stretcher should be carried by four bearers. As the first aider in charge, decide on the carrying method and give clear instructions to the bearers. After the casualty has been strapped to the stretcher, position yourself so you can watch the casualty and at the same time give direction to the other bearers.

Assign the remaining bearers (depending whether you are two or four) to respective corners or ends of the stretcher. Bearers crouch by the carrying handles of the stretcher, facing in the direction of travel.

- When the bearers have a firm footing and a good grip on the stretcher, give the command, "Get ready to lift," and then, "Lift."

- Ask the bearers if they are ready. When they are, give the command, "Go forward."

- When it is necessary to stop, give the commands "Stop," Get ready to lower," and then, "Lower."

To ensure the smoothest carry for the casualty:

- four bearers carrying a stretcher step off together on the foot nearest the stretcher and keep in step

- two bearers step off on opposite feet and walk out-of-step

Although stretcher casualties are usually carried feet first, certain conditions call for a head-first carry:

- leg injuries during a long downhill carry or when descending stairs, a head-first carry decreases pressure on the lower limbs and minimizes discomfort

- uphill carries and going up stairs if there are no injuries to the legs—a head-first carry decreases blood flow to the casualty's head and is more comfortable

- loading an ambulance or transferring the casualty to a bed—it is safer to do this head first, and easier to watch the casualty

2

Obstacles

When crossing uneven ground, a stretcher should be carried by four bearers and kept as level as possible. Bearers must adjust the height of the stretcher to compensate for dips and rises in the terrain.

Crossing a wall

Avoid crossing a wall, even if it means a longer carry. Where a wall must be crossed, follow these steps:

1. Lift the stretcher onto the wall so that the front handles are just over it. The rear bearers hold the stretcher level while the front bearers cross the wall. All lift together and the stretcher is moved forward until the rear handles rest on the wall.

2. The front bearers hold the stretcher level until the rear bearers have crossed the wall and resumed their positions at the rear of the stretcher.

3. The stretcher is then lowered to continue the journey.

Extrication

Extrication is the process of freeing casualties who are trapped or entangled in a vehicle or collapsed structure and cannot free themselves. Provide as much support as possible to the casualty during extrication. Whenever possible, give essential first aid and immobilize the injuries before the casualty is moved.

When there is an immediate danger and you are alone and must move a casualty from a vehicle, proceed as follows:

2

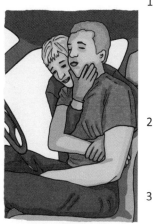

1   If necessary, disentangle the person's feet from the vehicle and bring the feet toward the exit. Ease your forearm under the person's armpit on the exit side, extending your hand to support the chin.

2   Ease the person's head gently backward to rest on your shoulder while keeping the neck as rigid as possible.

3   Ease your other forearm under the armpit on the opposite side and hold the wrist of the casualty's arm which is nearest the exit.

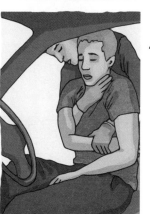

4   Establish a firm footing and swing around with the person, keeping as much rigidity in the neck as possible. Drag the casualty from the vehicle to a safe distance with as little twisting as possible.

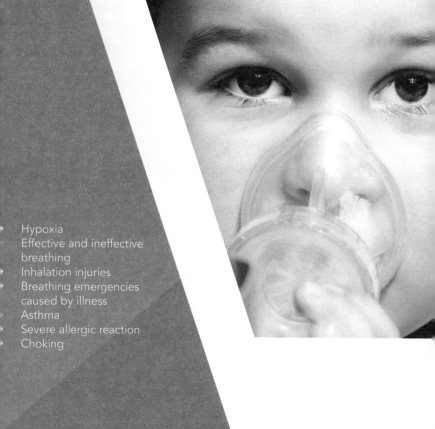

Airway and Breathing Emergencies

- Hypoxia
- Effective and ineffective breathing
- Inhalation injuries
- Breathing emergencies caused by illness
- Asthma
- Severe allergic reaction
- Choking

Chapter 3 Airway and breathing emergencies

When a person's breathing is affected through injury or illness, his life can be in immediate danger. As a first aider, you have to be able to recognize a breathing emergency very quickly and know what first aid to give—the casualty's life may depend on it.

3 Hypoxia

Choking and breathing emergencies cause a lack of oxygen in the blood, a condition called hypoxia. This can damage vital tissues and eventually cause death. The causes of hypoxia are grouped under three headings:

1.Lack of oxygen —for example:

- the oxygen level is low, such as at a high altitude
- the oxygen is displaced by other gases, such as a build-up of silo gas in a grain silo
- the oxygen in a small space is used up—for instance in a confined space

2.Blocked airway—for example:

- a casualty chokes on a foreign object, such as food
- an unconscious casualty's airway is blocked by their tongue
- a casualty's airway becomes swollen due to an allergic reaction

3.Abnormal heart and lung function—where the heart and lungs are not working properly due to:

- an illness such as pneumonia or congestive heart failure
- an injury preventing effective breathing
- a drug overdose or poisoning

Effective and ineffective breathing

The normal breathing rate varies for infants, children and adults. A breathing rate that is too slow or too fast is a sign of a breathing emergency. Breathing rhythm refers to the interval between breaths. In normal breathing, the intervals are even and breathing is effortless—this is regular breathing. Breathing depth refers to the amount of air moved in and out of the lungs with each breath. Signs of **effective breathing** include:

- breathing that is quiet
- equal expansion of both sides of the chest when the person inhales
- the person is alert and relaxed
- skin colour is normal
- speaking without taking a breath every few words

When a person is not getting enough oxygen, the body responds by breathing faster and deeper. Signs of **ineffective breathing** include:

- The casualty is struggling for breath or gasping for air
- Breathing rate is too fast or too slow
- Breathing rhythm is irregular
- Breathing depth is too shallow or too deep
- Breathing is noisy or raspy
- The person is "getting tired" from trying to breathe
- The person is sweating
- Decreased level of consciousness
- The lips, ears and fingernail beds turn blue—called cyanosis
- Chest movement may be abnormal

First aid for ineffective breathing

Always send or go for medical help at the first sign of a breathing emergency.

The first aid for ineffective breathing has two parts:

1. Give first aid for the injury or condition and position the responsive casualty in the semi-sitting position if possible

2. If breathing stops the casualty will become unresponsive, get medical help immediately and begin CPR

This table lists some of the causes of breathing emergencies. To give first aid, first determine the cause of the breathing emergency, and then decide on the best first aid actions.

Causes of airway and breathing emergencies		
Injuries	Medical conditions	Poisoning
broken ribs	asthma	inhaled poison – e.g. carbon monoxide or hydrogen sulfide
near drowning	stroke	swallowed poison – e.g. household cleaners or medication overdose
knife or gunshot wound	allergic reaction	injected poison – e.g. bee sting
burns to the face or airway	pneumonia	
head injury	congestive heart failure	
compression of the chest preventing chest expansion	emphysema/ bronchitis	

Inhalation injuries

Inhalation injuries happen when the casualty inhales hot steam or hot (superheated) air, smoke or poisonous chemicals.

Signs and symptoms of inhalation injuries include signs of shock:

- dizziness, restlessness, confusion
- pallor or cyanosis
- abnormal breathing rate or depth

Together with a history of fire and:

- noisy breathing
- pain during breathing
- burns on the face, especially the mouth and nose
- singed hair on the face or head
- sooty or smoky smell on breath
- sore throat, hoarseness, barking cough, difficulty swallowing

First aid for an inhalation injury

1. Perform a scene survey and do a primary survey. Give first aid for the ABCs.
2. Place a conscious casualty in the semi-sitting position and loosen tight clothing at the neck, chest and waist.
3. If breathing stops, begin CPR starting with compressions.
4. Give ongoing casualty care until handover to medical help.

Breathing emergencies caused by illness

Illnesses that can lead to severe breathing difficulties include asthma, allergies, chronic obstructive pulmonary disease (e.g. emphysema), congestive heart failure, stroke and pneumonia.

Asthma

Asthma is a reactive airway illness in which the person has repeated shortness of breath, characterized by wheezing and coughing. A mild asthma attack is not a health emergency and can be managed by the casualty. A severe asthma attack can be fatal and requires immediate first aid. In response to a 'trigger' the person's airway can spasm, swell and secrete thick mucus, which narrows the airway passage.

Some common triggers that can cause asthma are:

- colds, upper airway infections
- pet dander
- insect bites, stings
- foods
- pollen, paint and smoke

Signs and symptoms of a severe asthmatic attack:

- shortness of breath with obvious trouble breathing
- coughing or wheezing
- fast, shallow breathing
- casualty sitting upright trying to breathe
- bluish colour in the face (cyanosis)
- anxiety, tightness in the chest
- fast pulse rate, shock
- restlessness at first, and then fatigue

First aid for a severe asthma attack

1. Perform a scene survey and a primary survey; send for medical help.

2. Place the casualty in the most comfortable position for breathing. This is usually sitting upright with arms resting on a table.

3. Help the casualty take prescribed medication.

4. Give ongoing casualty care.

5. If the unconscious casualty stops breathing, begin CPR.

A person with asthma may carry medication in the form of a metered-dose inhaler (puffer). Usually the person can give himself this medication without help. If the person needs help, a first aider can assist.

An inhaler delivers a premeasured amount of medication. Always read and follow the manufacturer's instructions. Check the prescription label to confirm the casualty's name and expiry date.

1   Shake the container, then remove the cap.

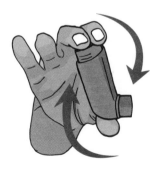

3

2   Tell the casualty to breathe out completely, then to breathe in slowly and deeply—as the casualty does, press the canister to release the medication. The canister can be in the mouth, or approximately four finger widths from the mouth.

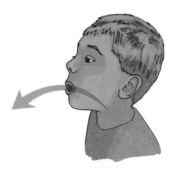

3   Tell the casualty to hold their breath for 10 seconds so the medication can spread out in the lungs. Then tell them to breathe normally, so the medication won't be expelled. If more doses are needed, wait at least 30-60 seconds before repeating these steps.

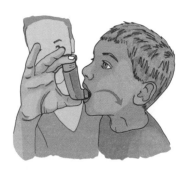

When the medication comes out of the inhaler, it may be deposited on the back of the throat and not reach the lungs or the casualty may be gasping for air and unable to hold their breath. To deal with this, use a spacer if available. It traps the particles of the spray, allowing the casualty to inhale more effectively over several breaths.

Spacers make it simple to inhale the medication, and should always be used when available. Small children and other casualties who have difficulties coordinating proper inhalation with the release of the medication will often have spacers with them.

3

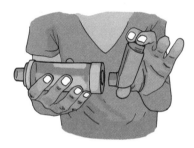

It allows them to inhale two or three times before the medication is completely dispelled. A mask can be attached to the device to make taking the medication easier.

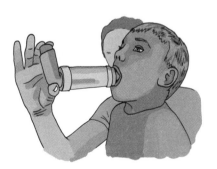

If the casualty complains of throat irritation after using the inhaler, have them gargle or rinse the mouth with water.

Severe allergic reaction

An allergic reaction occurs when the immune system reacts to a substance the body encounters. Most allergies are annoying but not dangerous.

Anaphylaxis is a severe allergic reaction which usually happens when a substance to which the casualty is very sensitive enters the body, although it can also be caused by exercise or have no known cause. Anaphylaxis can happen within seconds, minutes or hours of a substance entering the body. As a rule, the sooner the casualty's body reacts, the worse the reaction will be. Anaphylaxis is a serious medical emergency that needs urgent medical attention.

Common early **signs and symptoms** of an allergy may include itchy flushed skin with hives; sneezing and a runny nose; coughing. If it's a severe reaction there may be swelling of the face and neck, especially the lips and tongue. Breathing may become difficult if the swelling is internal too. There may be nausea and vomiting and the casualty may be anxious and feeling sense of impending doom as their blood pressure drops and they go into shock. This is a true medical emergency and requires immediate first aid.

First aid for a severe allergic reaction

1. Perform a scene survey and a primary survey. Send for medical help.
2. Place the casualty in the most comfortable position for breathing—usually sitting upright.
3. Assist the casualty with their medication, usually this is an epinephrine autoinjector.
4. Give ongoing casualty care.

How to help with medication for anaphylaxis

Anaphylaxis medication (epinephrine) is injected into the body with a needle. The use of EpiPen® Auto-injector is explained here. This device is designed for simple use and gives the right amount of medication with each injection. If the casualty cannot give the injection to himself, the first aider is permitted to use the autoinjector on the casualty. This includes an unconscious casualty where the first aider is certain of the cause. The effects of the medication may wear off. If a second dose is available, you may need to assist with it.

Auto-injectors are disposable drug-delivery systems with a spring-activated, concealed needle. It is important to be familiar with, and follow the manufacturer's instructions.

An auto-injector delivers a single dose of medication. A casualty may have more than one auto-injector for multiple doses.

3

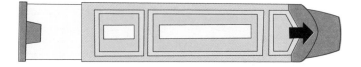

It is important to be familiar with, and follow the manufacturer's instructions, which is located on the side of the auto-injector.

Check the expiry date. If the only auto-injector is an expired product, it may still save a life and should be administered anyway, if the indicated liquid remains clear.

To use the auto-injector:

1. Remove the EpiPen® from the storage tube. Hold it firmly with the orange tip downward. Remove the blue safety release.

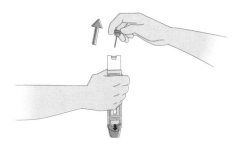

2. Only use the auto-injector on the fleshy part of the mid-outer thigh. Auto-injectors can be given through lightweight clothing. Press the orange tip of the EpiPen® firmly into the mid-outer thigh until the unit activates. Hold the auto-injector in place for several seconds, then pull it straight out.

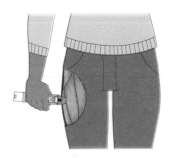

3. After the injection, keep the casualty warm and avoid any exertion. Call 9-1-1 as soon as you have given the first dose. If the casualty shows no improvement within 5 minutes or if their condition deteriorates before help arrives a second dose may be given if it is available. This will require a second EpiPen®. Individuals who are feeling faint or dizzy because of impending shock should be placed flat on their back unless they are vomiting or experiencing respiratory distress. It is important that the casualty does not sit or stand immediately as this could cause a drop in blood pressure. The medication will begin to wear off within 10 to 20 minutes—get medical help right away.

3

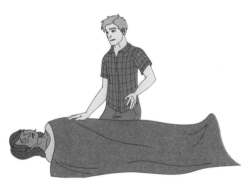

If you or anyone else is injected by mistake, get medical help.

Follow manufacturer's directions for proper care of the used device. Put the used unit back in the storage container and take it to the hospital with the casualty.

Choking

A person chokes when the airway is partly or completely blocked and airflow to the lungs is reduced or cut off. The choking casualty either has trouble breathing or cannot breathe at all.

Open and clear airway

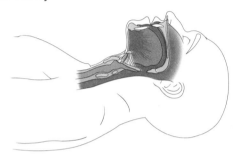

Partly blocked airway

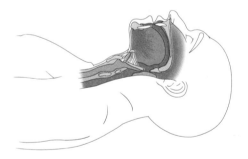

Completely blocked airway

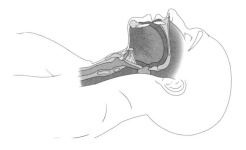

3

Causes of choking

Foreign objects	The tongue	Swelling
infants and children—food, toys, buttons, coins, etc.	tongue falls to the back of the throat when lying on back	injury to the throat area causes swelling of the airway
adults—consuming drinks quickly with food in your mouth	saliva, blood or vomit pools in the throat	illness causes swelling, e.g. allergic reaction, asthma, epiglottitis, croup
in elderly people—food, pills		Swollen airway

With good air exchange, the obstruction is mild and person can still cough forcefully, breathe and speak. With poor air exchange, the obstruction is severe and the person cannot cough forcefully, has trouble breathing, or cannot speak. With a completely blocked airway, there is no air exchange—coughing, breathing and speaking are impossible.

When the air supply to the lungs is cut off, the person's face immediately becomes red or "flushed". Shortly after, as the oxygen in the body is used up, the face becomes grey and the lips and ear lobes become blue. The person then becomes unconscious and eventually the heart stops beating.

Signs of choking	
Mild obstruction	**Severe obstruction**
able to speak	not able to speak
signs of distress—eyes show fear	signs of distress—eyes show fear
forceful coughing	weak or no coughing
wheezing and gagging between coughs	high-pitched noise or no noise when trying to breathe
red or "flushed" face	grey face and blue lips and ears

3

First aid for choking

First aid for a choking adult or child

1. Perform a scene survey.

2. If the casualty can cough forcefully, speak or breathe, tell them to try to cough up the object. If a mild obstruction lasts for a few minutes, get medical help.
   If you think there might be a severe obstruction, check by asking, "Are you choking?" If the casualty cannot cough forcefully, speak or breathe, use back blows followed by abdominal thrusts to remove the blockage.

3. Give back blows and abdominal thrusts:

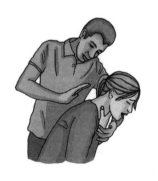

- Support the casualty and give up to five blows between the shoulder blades using the heel of your hand.

- If the obstruction is not cleared, step behind the casualty ready to support them if they become unconscious.

- Make a fist, place it on the casualty's abdomen at the belly button, in line with the hip bones. Grasp the fist with the other hand and give five forceful inward and upward abdominal thrusts.

4. If the object is not removed, repeat back blows and abdominal thrusts.

5. If the casualty becomes unconscious, lower them to the ground. Call for medical help and get an AED if available.

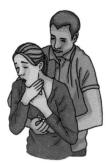

6. Begin chest compressions immediately. After the first 30 compressions, check the mouth. Remove any foreign object you can see. Try to give 2 breaths. If air does not go in, continue to give chest compressions and inspecting the mouth before ventilations.

First aid for a choking casualty much larger than the rescuer

If a choking casualty is very large or is in the late stages of pregnancy, give back blows as normal, followed by chest thrusts.

1. While supporting the casualty, give up to five back blows between the shoulder blades, using the heel of your hand.

2. If the obstruction is not cleared, stand behind the casualty.

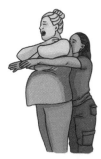

3. Keep your arms horizontal and snug up under their armpits.

4. Place your fist against the lower half of the breastbone, thumb-side in.

5. Hold your fist with your other hand. Pull inward forcefully.

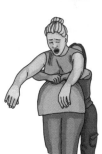

6. Continue giving back blows and chest thrusts until either the object is removed or the casualty becomes unconscious.

Choking adult – self-help

If you begin to choke on an object you may have to clear your own airway.

1. If there are people around, get their attention, do not isolate yourself from others.
2. Try to cough up the object.
3. Give yourself abdominal thrusts until you can cough forcefully, breathe or speak.

A second method is to use a solid object like the back of a chair, a table or the edge of a counter.

- Position yourself so the object is just above your hips.
- Press forcefully to produce an abdominal thrust.

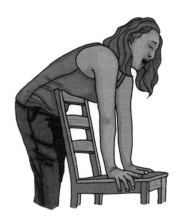

How abdominal thrusts work

When you choke on something, your body tries to unblock your airway by coughing.

Abdominal thrusts try to do the same thing with an artificial cough. The illustration below shows how an abdominal thrust creates a cough.

3

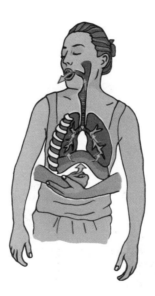

An abdominal thrust pushes the diaphragm up towards the lungs very quickly. This forces the air from the lungs up the airway and hopefully blows the obstruction out.

For the best effect, the fist has to be in the correct place. Keep your forearms off the abdomen and make each thrust a strong and sudden movement.

First aid for a choking casualty in a wheelchair

If you can reach around from behind the wheelchair, give back blows as normal, and abdominal or chest thrusts. If you cannot reach around the wheelchair:

- Position the wheelchair against a wall.
- Put the wheelchair brake on.

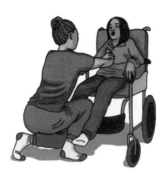

- If possible, carefully lean the casualty forward and support the shoulders. Perform five back blows between the shoulder blades, using the heel of your hand.
- Put the heel of one hand, with the other on top, in the middle of the abdomen and give up to five sudden, inward/upward thrusts.
- Alternatively, place the heel of one hand on the center of the breastbone and give firm chest thrusts.
- Repeat back blows and abdominal or chest thrusts until the object is removed or the casualty becomes unconscious.

If a doctor, physiotherapist or other health professional has shown you a different way of giving abdominal thrusts to a person in your care, use the recommended method.

If the casualty becomes unconscious, take them out of the wheelchair.

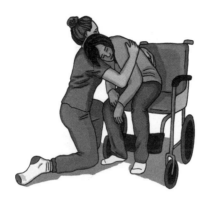

- Call for medical help and get an AED.

- Pull the casualty forward supporting them as best as you can and lower them to the ground.

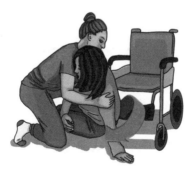

- Roll the casualty to the floor to a face-up position.

- Begin chest compressions immediately. After the first 30 compressions, check the mouth. Remove any foreign object you can see. Try to give 2 breaths and continue to give chest compressions and inspecting the mouth before ventilations.

First aid for a choking infant

An infant is choking when they suddenly have trouble breathing, coughing, gagging, with high-pitched, noisy breathing.

1. Perform a scene survey and primary survey.

2. If the baby can cough forcefully or breathe let the baby try to cough up the object. If a mild obstruction lasts for more than a few minutes, send for medical help.

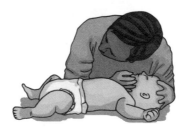

3. If the baby cannot cough forcefully, cannot breathe, makes a high-pitched noise when trying to breathe or starts to turn blue, begin back blows and chest thrusts.

4. Secure the baby between your forearms and turn them face down.

5. With the baby's head lower than the body, use the heel of your hand to give five forceful back blows between the shoulder blades.

6. Turn the baby face-up and give five chest thrusts.

7. Keep giving back blows and chest thrusts until either the airway is cleared or the baby becomes unconscious.

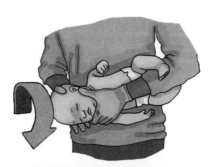

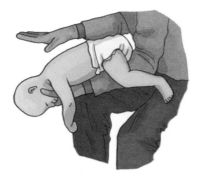

3

8. If the baby becomes unconscious, send for medical help. Begin chest compressions immediately.

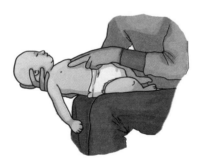

After the first 30 compressions, check the mouth. Remove any foreign object you can see. Try to give 2 breaths and continue to give chest compressions and inspecting the mouth before ventilations

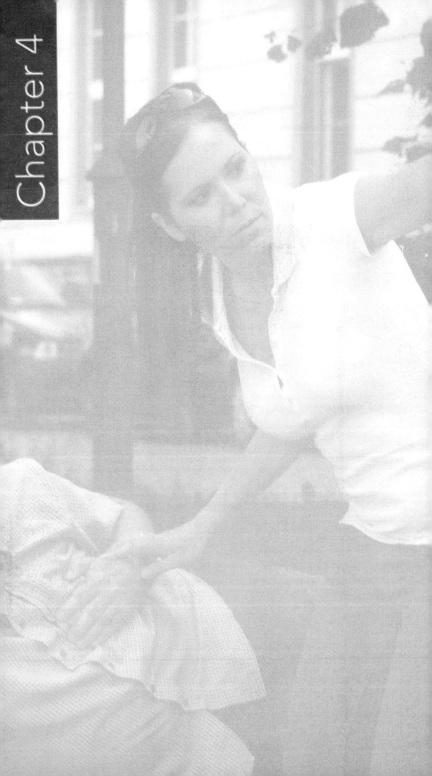

Cardiovascular Emergencies and Cardiopulmonary Resuscitation (CPR)

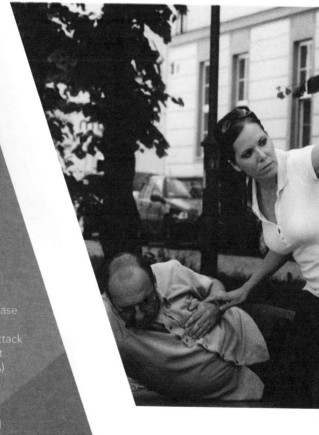

Cardiovascular disease
Chain of survival
Angina and heart attack
Stroke and transient
ischemic attack (TIA)
Cardiac arrest
Cardiopulmonary
resuscitation (CPR)
Automated external
defibrillation - (AED)

Chapter 4 Cardiovascular emergencies and Cardiopulmonary Resuscitation (CPR)

Cardiovascular disease

Cardiovascular disease is one of the leading causes of death of adults in Canada. Some of these deaths could be prevented if appropriate first aid was given. This chapter describes the first aid for cardiovascular emergencies, including

4

- first aid for angina/heart attack
- first aid for cardiac arrest, which is CPR
- first aid for stroke/TIA

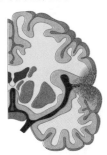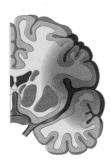

Angina

Angina occurs when the blood supply feeding the heart muscle becomes limited due to narrowed, damaged, or blocked arteries. When the heart works harder and needs more blood (e.g. when you run for a bus or shovel snow), it cannot get enough blood. This causes pain or discomfort in the chest, which may spread to the neck, jaw, shoulders, and arms. Angina pain typically doesn't last long, and goes away if the person rests and takes their prescribed medication.

Heart attack

A heart attack happens when heart muscle tissue dies because its supply of blood has been cut off. A heart attack can feel just like angina, except the pain doesn't go away with rest and medication. If the heart attack damages the heart's electrical system, or if a lot of the heart muscle is affected, the heart may stop beating properly. This is cardiac arrest.

Cardiac arrest

Cardiac arrest means the heart stops beating properly. With no blood flow going to the brain the casualty becomes unresponsive and stops breathing. Cardiac arrest means the casualty is clinically dead, but if CPR is started and a defibrillator is applied quickly there is still an opportunity to restore a normal heartbeat.

Stroke

A stroke happens when blood flow to a part of the brain is interrupted either by a blocked artery or by a ruptured blood vessel in the brain. A stroke may cause brain damage which impairs certain body functions, depending on the part of the brain affected.

Transient ischemic attack (TIA)

A TIA is a temporary blockage of the blood flow to part of the brain. It's typically of short duration and leaves no permanent damage but looks exactly like a stroke.

Doctors now have therapies to restore blood flow to the heart muscle and brain, but they work best if used right away. This is why it's important to realize there's an emergency and call 9-1-1 to get the casualty to the hospital right away—the longer medical help is delayed, the more likely the heart or the brain will be damaged.

4

Chain of Survival®

CPR is often what comes to mind when people think of first aid for a heart attack or cardiac arrest. But CPR is only part of the picture. There are five steps that are important when helping someone with heart problems.

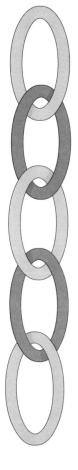

1. Immediate recognition of a cardiovascular emergency and activation of the community emergency medical services (EMS) system. This means calling for help quickly.

2. Early CPR with an emphasis on chest compressions.

3. Rapid defibrillation.

4. Effective advanced life support.

5. Integrated post-cardiac arrest care.

Each of the steps is as important as the others. Time is a vital ingredient. To give a casualty in cardiac arrest a reasonable chance of survival, CPR must be started immediately followed by defibrillation as quickly as possible. For both procedures, the sooner they happen, the better.

You, the first trained person on the scene, are responsible for initiating the sequence. You must recognize the cardiovascular emergency, call for medical help, start CPR if needed, and apply a defibrillator if one is available. You are the crucial first three links in the Chain of Survival®.

4

Angina and heart attack

Early recognition and denial

The first step is recognizing a cardiovascular emergency. It's difficult to accept that someone is having a heart attack and could die very soon, especially if the person is a family member or a close friend. The casualty is often denying anything serious is happening as well, so it's easy to accept their reassurances.

On average, casualties take several hours to get to a hospital from the time they first start feeling poorly. It is this wasted time that prevents many lives from being saved. When someone complains of chest pain, shortness of breath and looks odd you should consider it a serious problem—that's early recognition, and call for medical help. Getting the casualty to the hospital quickly gives them the best chance for survival. If nothing is wrong the ambulance crew can reassure the casualty. On the other hand, if there is a serious problem, you may have saved a life.

4

Signs and symptoms of angina and a heart attack:

A heart attack will produce shock and may display some or all of the following:

- pale, ashen skin

- sweating, cold and clammy to the touch

- shortness of breath

- showing obvious pain or discomfort

The pain or discomfort will be in the upper body, from the upper abdomen to the jaw and arms, and may feel like:

- heaviness in chest
- tightness or pressure in chest
- squeezing or crushing chest
- indigestion, nausea or vomiting
- aching jaw
- sore shoulder or arms

Some other **signs and symptoms** include:

- fatigue
- anxiety, which produces denial
- central back pain

Denial is an important detail. If someone showing signs of shock, having trouble breathing and experiencing pain insists there is nothing wrong, then you should be very suspicious and take action.

First aid for angina/heart attack

1. Perform a scene survey, then do a primary survey. Ask the casualty questions :
   "Can you show me where it hurts?"

   "Have you had this pain before?"

   "Do you have medication for this pain?"

2. Call for medical help and get a defibrillator.

3. Place the casualty at rest, the semi-sitting position is usually the best option, and reassure them.

4. Assist the conscious casualty to take their prescribed medication, usually nitroglycerin. If the casualty has no prescribed medication, or the first dose is ineffective, ask the casualty if they have any allergies to ASA, or if a doctor has ever told them not to take it. If the casualty believes they can take it, suggest they chew one regular ASA tablet (or two low-dose tablets). ASA can reduce the effects of a heart attack because of its anti-clotting properties.

5. If the casualty loses consciousness and stops breathing, start CPR.

Helping with Nitroglycerin

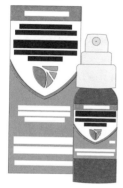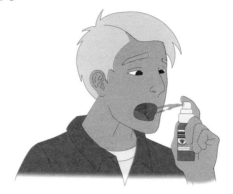

Nitroglycerin tablets or sprays are common medications for relief of chronic angina pain. A casualty in serious distress may need your help to take their medication.

Ask the casualty if they have taken any other medications today. Drugs to treat erectile dysfunction such as Viagra® or CIALIS® may cause a significant decrease in the person's blood pressure if nitroglycerin is taken as well.

Have the casualty spray the medication under the tongue or place the tablets under the tongue—they aren't to be swallowed. Nitroglycerin may be repeated, if needed, every 5-10 minutes to relieve pain, or until a maximum of three doses have been taken. Remember that if you have to assist someone to take their medication, you must call for medical help!

Stroke and transient ischemic attack (TIA)

A stroke or cerebrovascular accident (CVA) happens when a cerebral artery is blocked, usually by a blood clot, (an ischemic stroke) or a cerebral artery ruptures (a hemorrhagic stroke). A severe stroke can cause death; a less severe stroke may cause brain damage, which impairs certain body functions, depending on the part of the brain affected.

A transient ischemic attack (TIA) is caused by a lack of oxygen to part of the brain. It has the same signs and symptoms as a stroke but usually lasts from a few minutes to several hours and leaves no permanent brain damage. Advise anyone who has a TIA to get medical help.

Remember FAST as a way to check for the **signs and symptoms** of a stroke and to get immediate help.

- Facial droop. Ask them to smile. One side of the face may not move as well as the other side.

- Arm drift. Ask the casualty to hold both arms out with the palms up, and close their eyes. One arm may not move or drifts down compared to the other arm.

- Speech. Ask them to repeat a phrase you say. The casualty may slur words, use the incorrect words or is not able to speak.

- Time. When was the onset of symptoms? Ask the casualty, or their family, friends, or bystanders when the symptoms were first noticed. Get immediate medical help; the earlier a stroke is treated the better the outcome.

First aid for stroke/TIA

1. Perform a scene survey, then do a primary survey; perform the FAST assessment.

2. Call for medical help.

3. Place the casualty at rest in the semi-sitting position.

4. Give nothing by mouth, especially ASA.

5. Give ongoing care.

If the casualty becomes unconscious, place them in the recovery position. If there is paralysis, position the casualty with the paralyzed side up. This will reduce the chance of tissue or nerve damage to the affected side.

Cardiac arrest

When the heart stops pumping blood properly, it is called cardiac arrest, and the casualty is considered clinically dead, though they may still be resuscitated. The first aid for cardiac arrest is cardiopulmonary resuscitation (CPR) and rapid defibrillation.

Cardiopulmonary Resuscitation (CPR)

CPR is artificial respiration and artificial circulation. Artificial respiration provides oxygen to the lungs. Artificial circulation causes blood to flow through the body. The purpose of CPR is to circulate enough oxygenated blood to the brain and other organs to delay damage until either the heart starts beating again, or medical help takes over from you. CPR is most effective when interruptions to chest compressions are minimized.

4

CPR – Adult casualty

1. Perform a scene survey.

2. Assess responsiveness.

3. If there is no response, call for medical help on a mobile device, and place the phone on speakerphone, and send someone for an AED. If no mobile phone is available, send or go for medical help and the AED, if available. Perform a primary survey:

   Open the airway.

   Check for breathing for at least 5 and no more than 10 seconds.

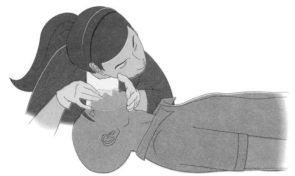

4. If the casualty is not breathing, or not breathing effectively (agonal breaths) position your hands in the centre of the upper chest and your shoulders directly over your hands. Keep your elbows locked.

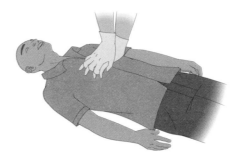

5. Give 30 compressions—Push hard—Push Fast!

- Press the heels of the hands straight down on the breastbone. The depth of each compression should be at 5-6 cm (2-2.4 inches).

- Release pressure and completely remove your weight at the top of each compression to allow chest to return to the resting position.

- Give compressions at a rate of 100 to 120 per minute. Count compressions out loud to keep track of how many you have given, and to help keep a steady rhythm.

6. Open the airway by tilting the head and lifting the chin.

7. Position a barrier device and breathe into the casualty twice. For an adult casualty, each breath should take about for 1 second, with just enough air to make the chest rise.

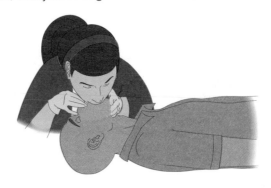

This is one cycle of 30:2 (30 compressions to 2 ventilations).

8. Continue CPR until either an AED is applied, the casualty begins to respond, another first aider or medical help takes over or you are too exhausted to continue. The AED should be applied as soon as it arrives at the scene.

Agonal breathing

Agonal breathing is an abnormal pattern of breathing driven by a brainstem reflex, characterized by irregular gasping respirations at times accompanied by strange vocalizations. They can occur with cardiac arrest and lead bystanders to believe the casualty is breathing. A casualty with agonal breathing should be treated as though they are not breathing.

4

CPR – Child casualty

1. Perform a scene survey.

2. Assess responsiveness.

3. If there is no response, send or call for medical help and an AED if available. If you are alone with no phone perform 5 cycles of CPR (two minutes) then go for mediacal help. Carry the child with you if possible. Perform a primary survey:

Open the airway.

Check for breathing for at least 5 and no more than 10 seconds.

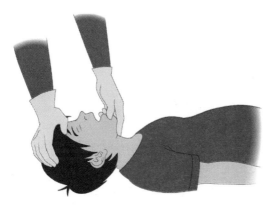

4. If the casualty is not breathing, or not breathing effectively (agonal breaths) position your hands in the centre of the upper chest and your shoulders directly over your hands. Keep your elbows locked. You may use one or two hands depending on the size of the child.

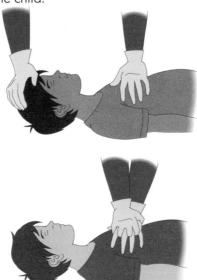

5. Give 30 compressions—Push hard—Push Fast!

- Press the heels of the hands straight down on the breastbone. The depth of each compression should be 1/3 of the chest depth, or 5 cm (2 inches).

- Release pressure and completely remove your weight at the top of each compression to allow chest to return to the resting position.

- Give compressions at a rate of 100 to 120 per minute. Count compressions out loud to keep track of how many you have given, and to help keep a steady rhythm.

6. Open the airway by tilting the head and lifting the chin.

7. Position a barrier device and breathe into the casualty twice, with just enough air to make the chest rise.

This is one cycle of 30:2 (30 compressions to 2 ventilations).

8. Continue CPR until either an AED is applied, the casualty begins to respond, another first aider or medical help takes over or you are too exhausted to continue. The AED should be applied as soon as it arrives to the scene.

CPR – infant casualty

1. Perform a scene survey.

2. Assess responsiveness. Gently tap the baby's feet.

If there is no response, call for medical help from a mobile device if possible, or, if you have no phone and no one to help, continue with the assessment and give 5 cycles of CPR if necessary (approximately 2 minutes) before calling for help.

Carry the infant with you to the telephone.

3. Open the airway. Check for breathing for at least 5 and no more 10 seconds.

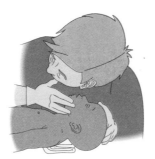

4. If the baby is not breathing, or not breathing effectively (agonal breaths) begin CPR

• Place two fingers on the breastbone just below the nipple line. Push down on the breastbone 1/3 the depth of the chest or about 4 cm (1 1/2 inches).

• Release the pressure completely but keep your fingers in light contact with the chest. Repeat the pressure and release phases rhythmically so that each phase takes the same amount of time.

• Give compressions at a rate of 100 to 120 per minute. Count compressions out loud to keep track of how many you have given, and to help keep a steady rhythm.

- Open the airway by tilting the head and lifting the chin.

  Position a barrier device and breathe into the casualty twice, with just enough air to make the chest rise.

Continue CPR until either an AED is applied, the casualty begins to respond, another first aider or medical help takes over or you are too exhausted to continue. The AED should be applied as soon as it arrives to the scene.

4

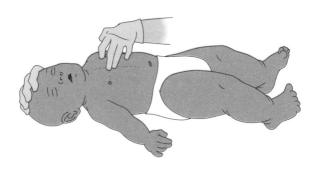

The back of an infant's head is quite large compared to the rest of the body. This causes the baby's head to come forward and close off their airway.

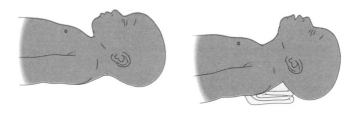

An infant's head flexes forward when they are lying on their back.

When giving CPR, it may be helpful to put a thin pad under the shoulders to help keep the airway open—but don't waste time looking for a pad.

Chest compression only CPR

CPR guidelines stress early recognition of the emergency and stress the importance of calling 9-1-1 or the local emergency number if you find someone collapsed and unresponsive.

If you have not been trained in CPR or are hesitant to perform ventilations, for any reason—don't give up. Your actions can still save a life.

Compression only CPR is CPR without mouth-to-mouth breaths. Provide high quality chest compressions by pushing hard and fast on the centre of the chest, at a rate of 100 to 120 compressions per minute.

4

Although this does not give the casualty any oxygen, this option can be used by people not trained in conventional CPR, or those who are unsure of their ability.

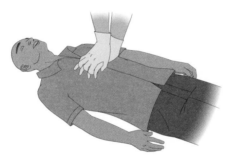

Dispatcher-assisted CPR

In many locales the 9-1-1 dispatcher is trained to coach you through an emergency until medical help arrives. Put your phone on speaker and place it by the casualty's head and talk to the dispatcher throughout the rescue.

How to take over CPR from another rescuer

1. Offer to help, tell the rescuer that you are trained in CPR. Ensure medical help has been called.

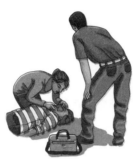

2. Give 30 compressions followed by 2 breaths. Use your own barrier device if available

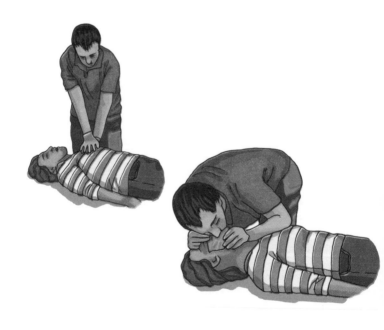

Two-rescuer CPR

If two trained rescuers are available, they can cooperate to perform CPR on a casualty. There are three advantages to two rescuers performing CPR as a team:

- CPR is a strenuous physical activity and as a first aider gets tired the quality of the chest compressions will deteriorate. By sharing the task of compressing the chest two rescuer CPR allows for a team to perform effective chest compressions for a longer period of time.

- Two-rescuer CPR minimizes the time the compressions are interrupted for ventilations to be given.

- Two-rescuer CPR allows the rescuers to give feedback and support each other during a stressful event.

To perform two-rescuer CPR the first aider who performs the primary survey stays at the casualty's head, keeping the airway open and ventilating after 30 compressions. The second rescuer will compress the chest, but in order to maintain the most effective compressions, it is recommended that rescuers switch after every 5 cycles of compressions and ventilations (approximately 2 minutes).

Automated External Defibrillation—AED

Automated external defibrillation, the application of an electric shock to a heart that has stopped pumping effectively, has been proven to be one of the most important tools in saving the lives of sudden cardiac arrest casualties. It is the third link in the Chain of Survival® and is the responsibility of the first aider.

An automated external defibrillator (AED) is an electronic device that is programmed to recognize and shock two types of heart rhythms, Ventricular Fibrillation (VF) and pulseless Ventricular Tachycardia (VT). If the machine recognizes either VT or VF in a casualty, it will charge and will indicate that a shock is advised. The purpose of this shock is to correct the abnormal electrical disturbance and re-establish the heart rhythm.

4

It is important to remember that AEDs will only shock when VT or VF is present. You cannot shock a heart that is in normal rhythm, nor will the machine shock when it is not appropriate, such as when the heart is stopping (asystole) or there is pulseless electrical activity (PEA)

Time is a critical factor in determining survival from cardiac arrest; the heart will only stay in fibrillation a short time before all electrical activity ceases. Defibrillation must be performed early to be most effective. CPR can keep oxygenated blood flowing to the brain, and helps extend the length of time that the heart will remain in VT or VF, the only arrhythmias that AEDs will shock. CPR then can "buy some time" for the casualty until the AED is attached and ready to deliver a shock.

Using an AED (always follow the AED's voice prompts)

1. Power on the AED.

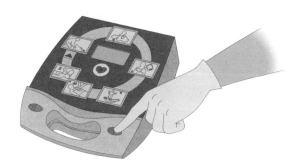

2. Follow the voice prompts. The audio instructions will direct you to:

- bare the chest and attach electrode pads. The pads need to stick directly to the skin, so excessive sweat, water, and chest hair needs to be removed before application

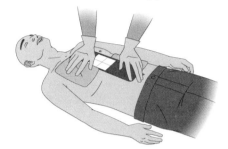

4

- stand back (or clear)

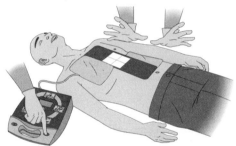

- press the shock button and/or continue CPR as prompted by the machine

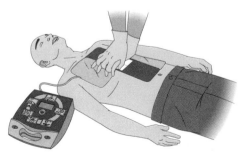

Continue with CPR and listen for the AED to give additional instructions

Defibrillation—Special Considerations and Special Circumstances

Pregnant patients—AEDs can be used in all stages of pregnancy.

Pacemakers or implanted defibrillators— Defibrillator pads should not be placed directly over a pacemaker site but should be approximately 2.5 cm (one inch) away. Look for scars or lumps on the chest as an indicator of implanted devices.

Children under 8 years of age—Automated external defibrillators (AEDs) may be used for children and infants. Special pads or a pediatric setting on the machine are used, but if not available adult pads can be used. Some adult pads show an alternate placement for children/infants.

Patch medications—some casualties wear a patch that contains medication such as nitroglyercin for angina. If the patch is in the way of the pad placement, gently remove it with gloved hands from the chest and wipe the area clean.

Wet environment—AEDs can be used in wet areas. Dry the chest to ensure good pad contact. Move the casualty to a dry area if possible. If you or the casualty is submersed in water, avoid using the AED.

Metal surfaces—AEDs can be used safely with the casualty on a metal surface.

Post-resuscitation care and handover to EMS

If defibrillation is successful, the casualty may start breathing on their own but remain unresponsive. In this case, place the casualty into the recovery position and monitor the ABCs. Leave the AED attached. The AED will continually monitor the heart rhythm or you may need to use the device again.

Certain information is important for emergency services personnel such as the time of collapse, time when CPR was started, time when first shock was delivered and number of shocks. Provide as much detail as possible and follow the directions of medical personnel once they arrive on the scene.

Troubleshooting and maintenance

Sometimes the device will indicate "Check Electrodes". If this occurs, check the cable to pads connection, the cable to machine connection and the adherence of the pads to the casualty's chest.

Machines will also advise if motion is detected or if the battery is low. AEDs are sold with an instruction manual that will outline troubleshooting in detail.

While AEDs are becoming easier to use and maintain, regular maintenance and operational checks are required and will help avoid problems when you have to use the device on a casualty. Follow the manufacturer's suggested schedule and checklist.

4

Chapter 5

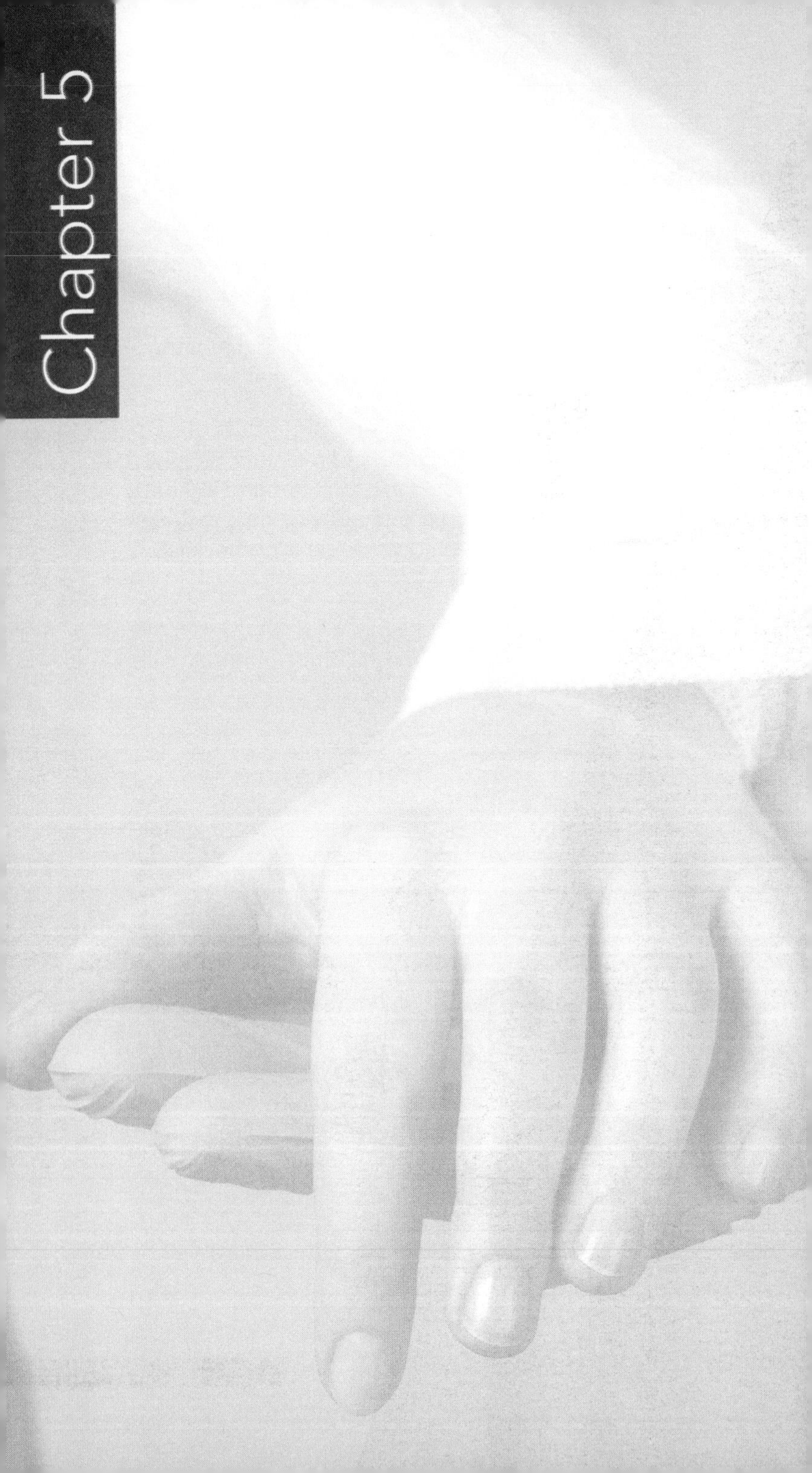

Wounds and
Bleeding

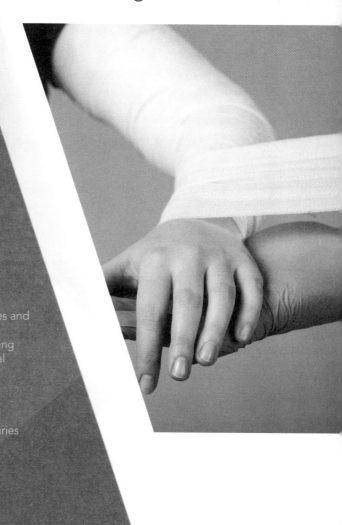

Chapter 5 Wounds and bleeding

Dressings, bandages, and slings

Dressings

A dressing is a protective covering put on a wound to help control bleeding, absorb blood from the wound, and prevent further contamination. A dressing should be:

- sterile, or as clean as possible
- large enough to cover the wound
- highly absorbent
- compressible, thick and soft
- non-stick and lint-free to reduce the possibility of sticking to the wound

Dressings are available in a variety of sizes and designs. The dressings used most often in first aid are:

- **adhesive dressings** – prepared sterile gauze dressings with their own adhesive strips

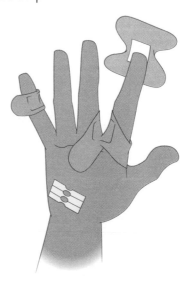

- **wound closures** – adhesive strips that bring the edges of the wound together to assist healing.

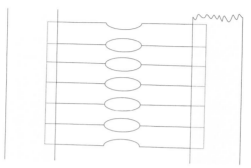

5

- **gauze dressings** – packaged gauze available as sterile single packs or in bulk packaging

- **pressure dressings** – large sterile dressings of gauze and other absorbent material, usually with an attached roller bandage. They are used to apply pressure to a wound with severe bleeding

- **improvised dressings** – prepared from lint-free sterile or clean absorbent material such as a sanitary pad

- **hemostatic dressings** – pressure dressings impregnated with clot promoting agents used to stop serious bleeding. These dressings are not designed for all wound types. Check with your local protocols for more information.

Follow the **guidelines** below for putting on dressings:

- prevent further contamination

- extend the dressing beyond the edges of the wound

- if blood soaks through a dressing, leave it in place and cover with more dressings

- secure a dressing with tape or bandages

Bandages

A bandage is any material that is used to hold a dressing in place, maintain pressure over a wound, support a limb or joint, immobilize parts of the body or secure a splint.

When using bandages, remember to:

- apply firmly to make sure bleeding is controlled or immobilization is achieved
- check the circulation below the injury before and after applying a bandage, you may have applied it too tightly or swelling may have made it too tight.

5

The triangular bandage

A triangular bandage may be used:

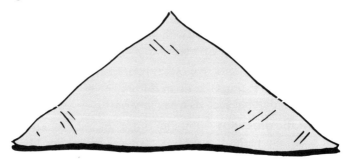

- as a whole cloth—opened to its fullest extent, as a sling or to hold a large dressing in place
- as a broad bandage—to hold splints in place or to apply pressure evenly over a large area
- as a narrow bandage—to secure dressings or splints or to immobilize ankles and feet in a figure-8

To form a broad bandage, fold the point to the centre of the base with the point slightly beyond the base

Fold in half again from the top to the base.

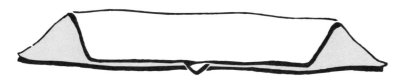

5

Fold a broad bandage in half again from the top to the base to form a narrow bandage.

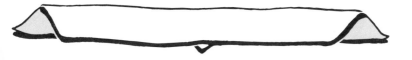

Reef knot—the knot of choice

The reef knot is the best knot for tying bandages and slings because:

- it lies flat, making it more comfortable than other knots
- it doesn't slip
- it is easy to untie in order to adjust the bandage

To tie a reef knot:

- take one end of a bandage in each hand
- lay the end from the right hand over the one from the left hand and pass it under to form a half-knot. This will transfer the ends from one hand to the other
- the end now in the left hand should be laid over the one from the right and passed under to form another half-knot. The finished knot looks like two intertwined loops
- tighten by pulling one loop against the other or by pulling only on the ends

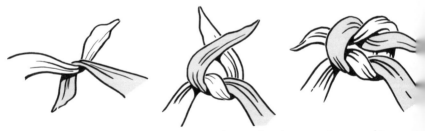

Place knots so they do not cause discomfort by pressing on skin or bone, particularly at the site of a fracture or at the neck, when tying a sling.

If the knot is uncomfortable, place soft material underneath as padding.

Figure-8

A figure-8 tie may be used to tie the ankles and feet, to secure a splint to the ankles/feet, or to support an injured ankle.

To tie a figure-8:

- Position the centre of a narrow or broad triangular bandage under the ankle (or both ankles if tying the feet together).

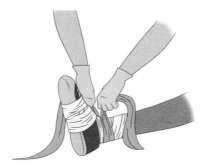

- Cross the ends over top the ankles, and bring the ends around the feet and tie off.

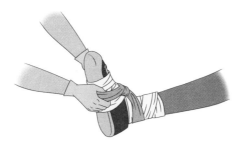

Roller bandage

Roller bandages, usually made of gauze-like elastic material, are used to hold dressings in place or to secure splints.

Put on a roller bandage in a simple spiral. Starting at the narrow part of the limb, anchor the bandage with a few turns and continue wrapping the bandage, overlapping each turn by one quarter to one third of the bandage's width. Make full-width overlaps with the final two or three turns and secure with a safety pin, adhesive tape or by cutting and tying the bandage as shown. Always check circulation below the wound before and after applying a bandage, you may have applied it too tightly or swelling may have made it too tight.

5

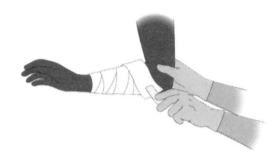

Slings

A sling can be easily improvised with a scarf, belt, necktie or other item that can go around the casualty's neck. You can also support the arm by placing the hand inside a buttoned jacket or by pinning the sleeve of a shirt or jacket to the clothing in the proper position.

Arm sling

To put on an arm sling:

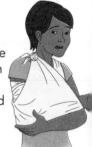

1. Support the forearm of the injured limb across the body. Place an open triangular bandage between the forearm and the chest so the point extends beyond the elbow and the base is straight up and down.

2. Bring the upper end around the back of the neck to the front of the injured side. While still supporting the forearm, bring the lower end of the bandage over the hand and forearm and tie off on the injured side in the hollow of the collarbone. Place padding under the knot for comfort.

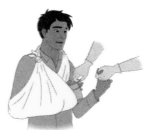

3. Twist the point into a "pigtail" at the elbow and tuck it inside the sling.

4. Adjust the sling so you can see the fingernails—this way you can watch them to check on circulation.

St. John tubular sling

This sling is used for injuries to the shoulder or collarbone. To put on a St. John tubular sling:

1. Support the forearm of the injured side diagonally across the chest, the fingers pointing toward the opposite shoulder.

2. Place a triangular bandage over the forearm and hand with the point extending beyond the elbow and the upper end over the shoulder on the uninjured side. The base is placed vertically in line with the body on the uninjured side.

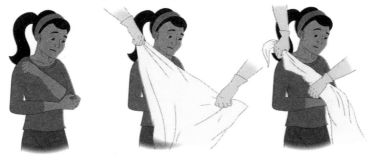

3. Ease the base of the bandage under the hand, forearm and elbow. Tuck the base of the bandage under the injured arm to make a pocket that runs the full length of the arm.

4. Gather the bandage at the elbow by twisting it and bring the lower end across the back and over the shoulder on the

uninjured side. This closes the pocket at the elbow.

5. Gently adjust the height of the arm as you tie off the ends of the bandage so the knot rests in the natural hollow above the collarbone. Place padding under knot, if available. Tie the sling tightly enough to support the weight of the injured arm.

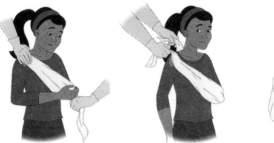
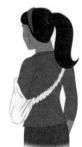

5

Wounds and bleeding

A wound is any damage to the soft tissues of the body. It usually results in the escape of blood from the blood vessels into surrounding tissues, body cavities or out of the body.

A wound can be either open or closed:

- **open wound**—a break in the outer layer of the skin
- **closed wound**—no break in the outer layer of skin but there is internal bleeding

The aim in the care of wounds is to stop the bleeding and prevent infection. Although some bleeding may help to wash contamination from the wound, excessive blood flow must be stopped quickly to minimize shock.

5

Types of wounds

Contusions or bruises

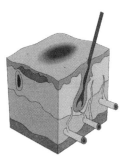

Contusions or bruises are closed wounds. The tissues under the skin are damaged and bleed into surrounding tissues, causing discolouration. A bruise may be a sign of a deeper, more serious injury or illness.

Abrasions or scrapes

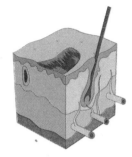

5 Abrasions or scrapes are open wounds where the outer protective layer of skin and the tiny underlying blood vessels are damaged. The deeper layer of the skin is still intact.

Incisions

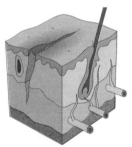

Incisions are clean cuts caused by something sharp such as a knife.

Lacerations

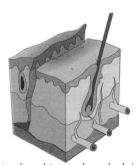

Lacerations are tears in the skin and underlying tissue with jagged and irregular edges.

Puncture wounds

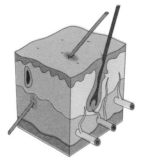

Puncture wounds are open wounds caused by blunt or pointed instruments that may have a small opening, but often penetrate deep into the tissue.

Avulsions and Amputations

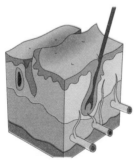

Avulsions are injuries that leave a piece of skin or other tissue either partially or completely torn away from the body.

Amputations involve partial or complete loss of a body part.

5

Bleeding

Bleeding is the escape of blood from the blood vessels. In external bleeding, blood escapes the body through a surface wound. In internal bleeding, blood escapes from tissues inside the body.

In arterial bleeding, the blood is bright red and spurts with each heartbeat.

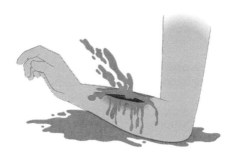

In venous bleeding, the blood is dark red and flows more steadily.

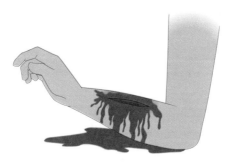

Severe blood loss will result in the following **signs and symptoms** of shock:

- pale, cold and clammy skin
- rapid pulse, gradually becoming weaker
- faintness, dizziness, thirst and nausea
- restlessness and apprehension
- shallow breathing, yawning, sighing and gasping for air

First aid for severe external bleeding

1. Perform a scene survey, then do a primary survey.

2. To control severe bleeding, apply direct pressure to the wound.

3. Place the casualty at rest.

4. Once bleeding is under control, continue the primary survey, looking for other life-threatening injuries.

5. Before bandaging the wound, check circulation below the injury. Bandage the dressing in place.

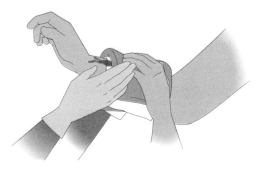

6. Check the circulation below the injury and compare it with the other side. If it is worse than it was before the injury was bandaged, loosen the bandage just enough to improve circulation if possible.

7. Give ongoing casualty care.

If the dressings become blood-soaked, don't remove them—add more dressings and continue pressure. Removing the blood-soaked dressings may disturb blood clots and expose the wound to further contamination.

Tourniquets and hemostatic dressings

For catastrophic wounds, where it will be difficult to control bleeding, the use of a tourniquet, a constricting bandage, to stop all blood flow to a limb, or hemostatic dressings to promote blood clotting may be considered. First aid kits for use by the military, law enforcement or wilderness first responders may contain specialized dressings or purpose built tourniquets to control bleeding.

Checking circulation below an injury

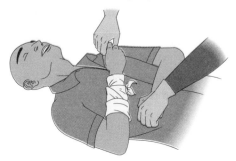

5

Injuries and first aid procedures may reduce or cut off circulation to the tissue below the injury (called distal circulation):

- Dislocations and fractures can impinge on an artery.

- Swelling or bandaging can compress an artery.

- Blood vessel damage may reduce blood flow through an artery.

If oxygenated blood does not reach the tissues below the injury, after several hours there may be tissue damage that could lead to loss of the limb. Check circulation below an injury before tying any bandages, then once again after tying the bandages. You may have applied the bandages too tightly or swelling may have made them too tight.

How to check circulation

Check circulation below the injury by comparing the injured limb to the uninjured limb:

- Check skin colour—if the skin does not have same colour as the uninjured side, circulation may be impaired.

- Check skin temperature—if the skin temperature feels colder than the uninjured side, circulation may be impaired.

- Check for a pulse—at the wrist or ankle, and compare to the other limb.

- Check the nail beds—press on a fingernail or toenail until the nail bed turns white, and then release it. Note how long it takes for normal colour to return, and compare to the uninjured side.

Improving impaired circulation

To improve impaired circulation:

- Loosen tight bandages.
- Reposition the limb to relieve any pressure on blood vessels in a fracture or dislocation. Only move the limb if there is no resistance or increased pain.

If circulation cannot be improved, get medical help immediately.

Preventing contamination

Minor wound care

All open wounds are contaminated to some degree. Tell the casualty to seek medical help if signs of infection appear later.

- Wash your hands with soap and water and put on gloves if available.
- Do not cough or breathe directly over the wound.
- Fully expose the wound but don't touch it.
- Gently wash loose material from the surface of the wound. Wash and dry the surrounding skin with clean dressings, wiping away from the wound. An antibiotic cream can be used on superficial wounds and abrasions.
- Cover the wound with a sterile dressing.

Wound infection

The acronym **SHARP** identifies signs and symptoms of infection.

S—**Swollen**

H—**Hot**, feels warmer than the surrounding area

A—**Aches**, a dull pain

R—**Red**

P—**Pus** may leak from the wound

Tetanus infection

Any wound may be contaminated by spores that cause tetanus, a potentially fatal bacterial disease characterized by muscle spasms. Tetanus is commonly referred to as "lockjaw."

Deep wounds are at especially high risk of tetanus infection. Advise a casualty with this type of wound to get medical help as soon as they can. Symptoms may not arrive immediately.

Recognizing internal bleeding

Suspect internal bleeding if:

5

- the casualty received a severe blow or a penetrating injury to the chest, neck, abdomen or groin

- there are major limb fractures such as a fractured upper leg or pelvis

Signs of internal bleeding:

- bleeding from the ear canal or the nose

- bloodshot or black eye (bleeding inside the head)

- coughing up blood that looks bright red and frothy (bleeding into the lungs)

- vomiting bright red blood, or brown blood that looks like coffee grounds

- blood in the stool that looks either red or black and tarry

- red or smoky brown-looking blood in the urine

- signs of shock with no signs of external injury

First aid for internal bleeding

1. Perform a scene survey. Have the casualty lie flat on their back and do a primary survey.

2. Send or go for medical help.

3. Give ongoing casualty care, including laying the casualty in the supine position, and giving first aid for shock.

You can do very little to control internal bleeding. Give first aid to minimize shock and get medical help as quickly as you can.

First aid for amputations

An amputation is when a part of the body has been partly or completely cut off. You must control the bleeding from the wound, care for the amputated tissue and get medical help.

1. Perform a scene survey, then do a primary survey.

2. Control bleeding—apply direct pressure to the wound. Reposition a partly amputated part to its normal position and bandage.

3. Send for medical help and continue ongoing casualty care to the casualty.

4. Care for the amputated part by wrapping it in a clean, moist

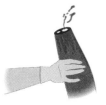 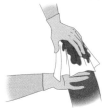

dressing (if clean water is available).

5. Put the amputated part in a clean, watertight plastic bag and seal it. Put this bag in a second plastic bag or container partly filled with crushed ice. Attach a record of the date and time this was done and send this package with the casualty to medical help.

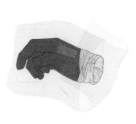 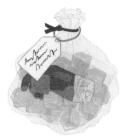

6. If direct pressure fails to control life-threatening external limb bleeding, a tourniquet could be considered by a trained first aider (in special circumstances, such as mass casualty management, a disaster, remote locations).

General first aid for hand and foot injuries

Hand and foot injuries are common. If the injury seems minor and the casualty chooses not to get medical help, instruct them to get medical help within 48 hours if there is still pain, loss of function, or an infection.

First aid for bleeding from the palm of the hand

1. Start ESM. Perform a scene survey.

2. Perform a primary survey and expose the wound.

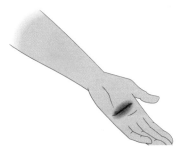

3. Control the bleeding with direct pressure with a bulky pad over sterile dressings. Check the circulation in the fingers and compare it with the other hand. Bend the fingers over the pad to make a fist and bandage the hand so the fist is held firmly closed:

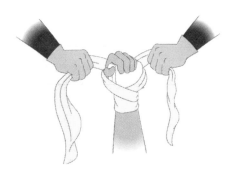

- Place the middle of a narrow triangular bandage on the inside of the wrist and bring the ends around the back of the hand, or start wrapping with a roller bandage at the wrist, and continue wrapping around the back of the hand.

- Wrap the tightly bandage over the fingers and then down around the wrist.

- Leave the thumb exposed, if possible, to check circulation. Tie the bandage off at the wrist and tuck in the ends.

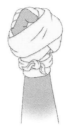

5

4. Give ongoing casualty care, recheck the circulation below the injury, and get medical help. Use a sling to support the arm and hand if transporting.

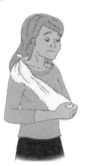

First aid for pinched fingernail

When a finger or toe nail has been pinched, sometimes called a nail bruise, the pressure from the blood under the nail can cause great pain. You can relieve this pain as follows:

- Place the injured part under cool running water to reduce pain and swelling.

- If the pain is severe, and you can see pooled blood under the nail, release the pressure under the nail as follows:

  - Straighten a paper clip or blunt wire and heat one end to red hot, using a stove element or the flame from a lighter. Don't use a needle, the hole it makes is too small to release the pooled blood effectively.

  - Place the heated end of the paper clip on top of the nail and let it melt a hole just deep enough to release the pooled blood.

  - Once the pressure has been released, wash the area with water and put on an adhesive dressing.

- Advise the casualty to seek medical help if signs and symptoms of an infection develop.

First aid for contusion (bruise)

With a contusion or bruise, blood escapes into the surrounding tissue. Relieve the pain and reduce the swelling by using the acronym **RICE:**

- Rest
- Immobilize
- Cold
- Elevate

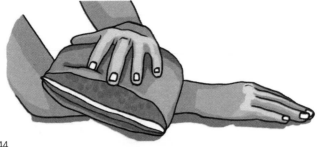

First aid for puncture wounds

Puncture wounds are serious because of the possibility of serious internal damage and contamination carried deep inside the wound.

1. Perform a scene survey. The mechanism of injury is important. Then perform a primary survey. Expose the wound. Although there may not be much external bleeding, you should suspect internal bleeding, especially if the wound is in the chest or abdomen.

2. Control bleeding with direct pressure on the wound, and get medical help.

3. Give ongoing casualty care until handover.

First aid for gunshot wounds

A gunshot wound is a serious type of puncture wound. The entry wound is often small, but the bullet may have travelled deep into or through the body and there may be an exit wound as well, which is often larger than the entry wound. The exit wound may not be directly across from the entry wound.

1. Perform a scene survey and ensure the area is safe for yourself and the casualty. Then perform a primary survey. Expose the wound and check carefully for an exit wound; it may not be where you expect it.

2. Control bleeding with direct pressure on the wound, and get medical help.

3. Place the casualty at rest and give first aid for shock.

4. Give ongoing casualty care.

First aid for wounds with embedded objects

Do not remove an object embedded in a wound if possible. Removing the object will probably result in heavier bleeding; the object can help stop bleeding. Removing it could cause further tissue damage too, for example a barb on a fish hook.

1. Expose the injured area and assess the wound. Check the circulation below the injury.

2. To stop the bleeding, put pressure around the embedded object. If the embedded object is short, "tent" a clean dressing loosely over the object to keep the wound clean, then place bulky dressings around the object to keep it from moving. This will apply pressure around the wound

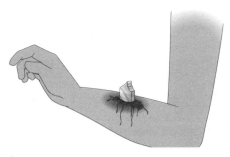

5

3. Secure the bulky material (dressings) in place with a narrow bandage, taking care that pressure is not exerted on the embedded object.

4. Check the circulation below the injury again.

5. Give ongoing casualty care and get medical help.

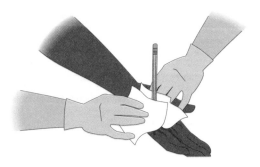

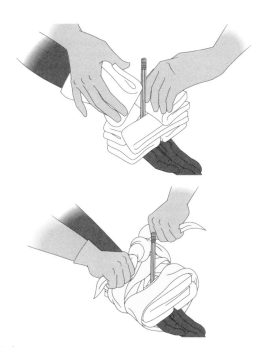

First aid for slivers and splinters

Slivers are small embedded objects - wood, thorns, glass or metal. This type of injury is common in the hands and feet. Although slivers may cause discomfort and pain, in most cases they can be removed easily without complications. In serious cases, slivers can be disabling and cause infection. Do not remove a sliver if it:

- lies over a joint
- is deeply embedded into the flesh
- is in or close to the eye
- has a barb (e.g. metal slivers and fishhooks)
- cannot be removed easily

In these cases, give first aid for an embedded object.

Removing a sliver

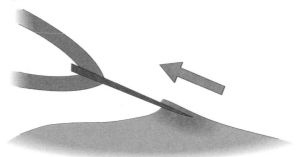

1. Clean the area with water.

2. With sterile tweezers, grip the sliver as close to the skin as possible.

3. Pull the sliver in a straight line in the opposite direction to the angle of entry.

4. Get medical help if some of the sliver was not removed, there is more tissue damage than a simple, small puncture wound or if an infection develops.

Chest injuries

Wounds to the chest can cause breathing problems and require immediate medical help.

Pneumothorax

A pneumothorax is caused by air in the chest between the lung and the chest wall. Air can enter from the outside, an open pneumothorax, or penetrating chest wound. Air can also enter from the lung, a closed (or spontaneous) pneumothorax. Breathing with a pneumothorax becomes impaired as the lungs begin to collapse. Medical help is required immediately.

First aid for a penetrating chest wound

1. Perform a scene survey and primary survey.

2. If the open chest wound has significant bleeding, cover it by pressing the casualty's hand, a bystander's hand or your own hand over the wound (preferably a gloved hand). If there is

no significant bleeding, the first aider may leave the wound exposed, or use a non-occlusive dressing. If the dressing becomes saturated, it must be changed.

3. Place the casualty in the position that makes breathing easiest—this is usually semi-sitting, leaning slightly towards the injured side. This position keeps the uninjured side of the chest upward so it can be used most effectively for breathing.

4. Do not seal the wound with an airtight dressing, but cover the wound to prevent further contamination. If the dressing becomes wet, replace it with a dry dressing.

5. Give ongoing casualty care, monitoring breathing often.

There is not always an open wound with a pneumothorax. A pneumothorax always has the potential to be a life-threatening breathing emergency and medical help is needed as quickly as possible.

First aid for a blast injury that affects breathing

For Canadians working in the mining and construction industries, explosives are a workplace hazard. There are three mechanisms of injury from an explosion:

• injuries from being struck by material thrown by the blast

• injuries from being thrown by the blast

• injuries to hollow organs, including the lungs, caused by the shock wave from the blast

The casualty may complain of chest pain and cough up frothy blood.

1. Perform a scene survey. If the casualty was thrown by the blast, suspect a head or spinal injury and prevent any unnecessary movement. Perform a primary survey.

2. Place the casualty in a semi sitting position if there is no suspected head or spinal injury. Send for medical help.

3. Monitor breathing closely.

4. Give ongoing casualty care.

Abdominal injuries

Abdominal wounds may be closed or open. Closed wounds occur when internal abdominal tissues are damaged but the skin is intact. An open abdominal wound has a break in the skin where internal organs may protrude. Complications from abdominal wounds may include severe bleeding (either internal or external) and contamination from the contents of ruptured abdominal organs.

To assess an abdominal injury expose the injured area and look for open wounds. Consider the history of the incident, especially the mechanism of injury. Observe the casualty's position; are they 'guarding' their abdomen? Gently feel for swelling, rigidity, and pain.

If you suspect an abdominal injury, you should also suspect **internal bleeding** that may be severe. Give first aid for severe internal bleeding.

First aid for open abdominal wounds

1. Perform a scene survey and a primary survey.

2. If you find an open abdominal wound you must be prevent it from opening wider. The internal organs may be displaced. Position the casualty in the semi-sitting position with the knees raised and supported.

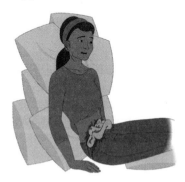

3. Dress the wound. The method of dressing a wound of the abdominal wall depends on whether or not internal organs are protruding:

- If the organs are not protruding, apply a dry dressing to the wound and bandage firmly.

- If the organs are protruding, do not try to put them back into the abdomen. Put on a moist dressing to stop the organs from drying out and bandage loosely with two broad bandages.

4. Give ongoing casualty care.

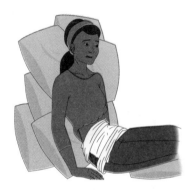

5

Crush injuries

A crushing force can cause extensive bruising of the area, and there may be complications including fractures or ruptured organs. When the crushed area is limited, such as a hand or foot, the injury is considered serious, but is not usually life-threatening. However, a major crush injury may cause **compartment syndrome**, and needs medical help immediately. This occurs when excessive pressure builds up inside the body, usually from bleeding or swelling after an injury. The dangerously high pressure in compartment syndrome can cut off the flow of blood through the affected area.

Severe shock can develop after a casualty is released from the weight that caused the crush injury. When the crushing force is removed, fluids from the crushed tissues leak into surrounding tissues—this causes shock.

When muscle is crushed, it releases the contents of muscle cells into the blood. If the injury is large, it can cause kidney failure. This is **crush syndrome**, also called post-traumatic acute renal (kidney) failure.

First aid for crush injuries

1. Perform a scene survey and a primary survey.

2. Give first aid for shock right away—even if there are no signs, shock will probably develop.

3. Call for medical help and give ongoing casualty care

Scalp and facial injuries

First aid for bleeding from the scalp

Bleeding from the scalp is often severe and may be complicated by a fracture of the skull or an embedded object. Avoid direct pressure, probing and contaminating the wound.

1. Perform a scene survey and a primary survey.

2. Apply a thick, sterile dressing and bandage it firmly in place with a head bandage.

3. If there is suspected underlying skull fracture, give first aid for a fracture of the skull.

4. If there is an embedded object, apply dressings around the object to maintain pressure around but away from the wound.

5. Give ongoing casualty care.

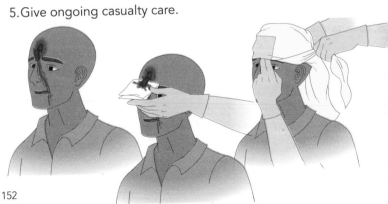

First aid for bleeding from inside the ear

Don't try to stop the bleeding from the ear canal by putting pressure on the ear or by packing it with dressings. To reduce the risk of infection inside the ear, it is best to let the blood drain away.

1. Perform a scene survey and assess the mechanism of injury. If you suspect a head or spinal injury, tell the casualty not to move. Do a primary survey.

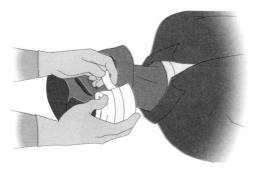

2. Assess the bleeding from the ear. If the blood from the ear is mixed with straw-coloured fluid, suspect a skull fracture— steady and support the head and neck. Place a dressing lightly over the ear and give first aid for a skull fracture. The dressing will absorb the blood and protect the wound.

3. If a head or spinal injury is not suspected, lightly tape a dressing over the ear. Position the casualty to allow the blood to drain from the ear if injuries permit. If the casualty is unconscious and injuries permit, put dressings over the ear and place them in the recovery position with the injured side down.

4. Give ongoing casualty care.

First aid for a nosebleed

A nosebleed may start for no obvious reason, or may be caused by blowing the nose, an injury to the nose, or by an indirect injury, such as a fractured skull.

1. Perform a scene survey and assess the mechanism of injury. If you suspect a head or spinal injury, tell the casualty not to move. Do a primary survey.

2. Assess the bleeding from the nose. If the blood from the nose is mixed with straw-coloured fluid, suspect a skull fracture. Allow the nose to bleed and give first aid for a skull fracture.

3. If a head or spinal injury is not suspected, place the casualty in a sitting position with the head slightly forward. Leaning forward allows blood to drain from the nose and mouth instead of back into the throat and stomach where it will cause vomiting.

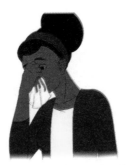

Tell the casualty to compress the entire fleshy part below the bridge of the nose firmly with the thumb and index finger for about 10 minutes or until bleeding stops.

4. Tell the casualty to breathe through the mouth and not blow their nose for a few hours, so that blood clots will not be disturbed. If bleeding does not stop with this first aid, or if it starts again, get medical help.

First aid for a knocked-out tooth

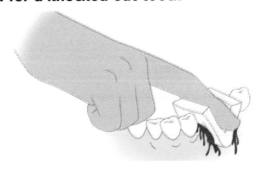

A knocked-out tooth can be re-implanted if the casualty receives medical/dental help quickly.

1. Perform a scene survey and assess the mechanism of injury. If you suspect a head or spinal injury, tell the casualty not to move. Do a primary survey.

2. Apply direct pressure to stop the bleeding from the socket of the tooth. Seat the casualty with the head forward so blood can drain out of the mouth.

3. Place the knocked-out tooth in a balanced salt solution, or coconut milk. If none of these are available, the casualties own saliva will do. Handle the tooth by the top—don't touch the root.

4. Give ongoing casualty care.

5

Bleeding from the cheek, gums or tongue

When there is bleeding from the gums or mouth, first assess the mechanism of injury to determine if there is a chance of a serious head and/or spinal injury. Make sure the bleeding in the mouth doesn't block the airway.

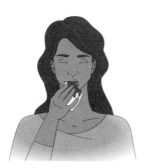

Control the bleeding in the mouth using direct pressure over a clean, preferably sterile, dressing. Do not wash out the mouth after bleeding has stopped, this may dislodge clots and cause bleeding to start again.

Eye injuries

The eye can be injured very easily; proper first aid given right away may prevent partial or complete loss of eyesight. Tears may not be enough to loosen and wash away irritating particles on the eye.

First aid for a loose foreign particle in the eye

1. Begin by asking the casualty where they feel the particle is located.

2. If it feels like the particle is under the upper lid, instruct the casualty to grasp the upper eyelashes and pull the lid straight out and then down over the lower eyelashes to try to sweep the particle away.

   Try this several times. Remember to remove excess eye make-up before attempting this procedure.

   If the particle is still in the eye, try flushing it out using clean running water from a tap, an eye cup or eye wash bottle.

   If the above methods have not been successful, you will need to examine the surface of the eye and under the lids.

Examining the eye

1. Seat the casualty facing a good light and steady the head.

2. Instruct the casualty to look to the left, right, up and down. A penlight directed across the eye will cause a shadow to appear if the particle is in the path of the light, making it easier to see.

3. To examine under the upper and lower lids, gently pull down on the lower lid and ask the casualty to look up. To examine under the upper lid, gently pull up on the lashes and ask the casualty to look down. Use your penlight to check under the lids.

4. If you locate the particle, remove it gently using the moist corner of a facial tissue, clean cloth or cotton-tipped applicator. Do not try to remove a particle that is stuck to the eye, or is located on the coloured part of the eye. If the casualty is wearing contact lenses, have them remove the lens before trying to remove a particle from the eye.

First aid when you cannot safely remove a particle from the eye

5

1. If removing the particle is unsuccessful, warn the casualty not to rub the eye because this may cause pain and tissue damage.

2. Close the casualty's eye and cover the affected eye with an eye or gauze pad. Extend the covering to the forehead and cheek to avoid pressure on the eye.

3. Secure lightly in position with a bandage or adhesive strips. Make sure there is no pressure on the eyeball.

4. Give ongoing casualty care and get medical help.

Wounds in the soft tissue around the eye

Wounds to the eyelid and soft tissue around the eye are serious because there may be injury to the eyeball. Blows from blunt objects may cause bruises and damage the bones that surround and protect the eyes.

Cover only the most seriously injured eye to avoid the psychological stress that the casualty may suffer when both eyes are covered. This leaves the casualty able to walk on their own. If both eyes must be covered due to serious injury, (e.g. intense light burn from arc welding), reassure the casualty often by explaining what is being done and why. This casualty must be carried.

First aid for lacerations and bruises around the eye

Lacerated eyelids usually bleed profusely because of their rich blood supply. A dressing on the area will usually control bleeding. Never apply pressure to the eyeball—this may force fluid out of the eyeball and cause permanent damage to the eye.

5

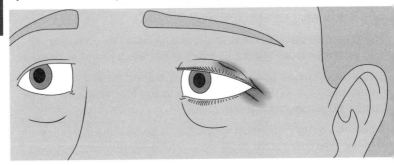

First aid for an embedded object in or near the eyeball

Give first aid for an embedded object in or near the eyeball. As for any embedded object, prevent the embedded object from moving since movement could cause further damage to the eyeball.

1. Perform a scene survey and primary survey. Have a bystander support the head.

2. Place dressings, preferably sterile, around the embedded object. Place padding or dressings around the object in a "log cabin" fashion, to stabilize the object. Make sure there is no pressure on the eyeball.

3. Arrange transportation of the casualty on a stretcher to medical help as soon as possible.

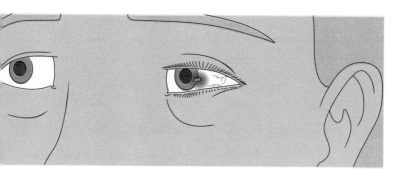

First aid for an extruded eyeball

"Extruded" means the eyeball has been thrust out of its socket. Do not try to put the eye back into position.

5

1. Perform a scene survey and primary survey. Have a bystander support the head.

2. Gently cover the eyeball and socket with a moist dressing. Hold this in place with tape and more dressings.

3. Give ongoing casualty care until handover.

First aid for chemical burns to the eye

The eyes can be permanently injured by corrosive chemicals in either solid or liquid form. Casualties normally suffer intense pain and are very sensitive to light. Give first aid as follows:

1. Perform a scene survey and primary survey. Have a bystander support the head.

2. Sit or lay the casualty down. If only one eye is injured, protect the uninjured eye.

3. If the chemical is a dry powder, brush away whatever is on the skin. Do not use your bare hands.

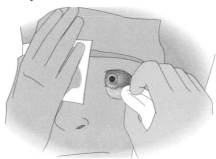

4. Flush the injured eye with cool water. Since pain may make it hard for the casualty to keep the eye open, gently open the eye with your fingers. Flush the eye for at least 15 minutes.

5. Cover the injured eye with dressings. If both eyes are injured, cover the more seriously injured eye. Only cover both eyes if the casualty is more comfortable that way. Covering both eyes blinds the casualty and adds to the stress of the scene. If you do cover both eyes, keep the casualty lying down.

6. Give ongoing casualty care.

If the casualty is wearing contact lenses

Don't waste time trying to remove contact lenses. Flush the eyes for 15 minutes—this may wash the lenses out. If not, have the casualty remove them. Lenses exposed to chemicals should be thrown away (so it doesn't matter if they are washed away during flushing).

When there is a risk of eye injury from chemicals, proper eye-wash equipment should be kept nearby.

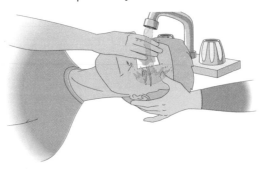

First aid for intense light burns to the eye

Burns to the eyes may be caused by prolonged exposure to intense light such as direct or reflected sunlight or a short duration event like the flash from an arc welder. Snow blindness is a common injury of this kind. As with a sunburn, the casualty may not feel the tissue damage happening but will develop symptoms several hours after exposure. Signs and symptoms include:

- sensitivity to light
- pain
- a gritty feeling in the eyes

Give first aid as follows:

1. Perform a scene survey and primary survey.
2. Cover the eyes to cool them and keep the light out. The casualty will be temporarily blinded, so reassure them often.
3. Give ongoing casualty care.

Burns

Burns are injuries to the skin and other tissues caused by heat, radiation or chemicals. They are a leading cause of injury in the home. Young children and elderly people are especially at risk of being burned, and at these ages, burn injuries can be serious.

Types of burns

Heat burns (also called "thermal" burns)

Burns from heat applied to the body are the most common of burns. A scald is a heat burn caused by hot liquid or steam. Heat burns can also be caused by friction.

5

Chemical burns

Chemical burns are often serious because the chemicals continue to burn as long as they remain on the skin. Examples of chemicals that can burn include acids or alkalis.

Electrical burns

5

Electrical burns result from contact with an electric current. Although it is heat that causes these burns, electrical burns are considered separately because of the complications caused by the electricity.

Radiation burns

Most people have experienced a radiation burn in the form of sunburn, where the sun is the source of radiant energy.

Other types of radiant energy that can cause burns include X-rays, arc welder's flash and radiation from radioactive material.

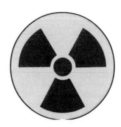

Severity of a burn

Burns are classified as **critical, moderate** or **mild** depending on:
- the depth of the burn
- the amount of body surface that is burned
- the part(s) of the body that is burned
- the age and physical condition of the casualty

Burn depth

The skin protects the body from bacteria, helps control body temperature and keeps body fluid in the body. When the skin is damaged by a burn, it cannot do these functions properly, or at all.

5

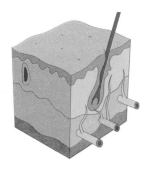

The severity of a burn depends on the depth of the tissue damage. The deeper the burn, the more serious it is. In first aid, burns are described as **superficial**, **partial thickness** or **full thickness** burns depending on how deep into the skin they extend.

Estimating the burned area—the rule of nines

A first aider can quickly estimate how much body surface area has been burned using the rule of nines. The body is divided up into areas of either nine or eighteen per cent of total body area. Add these areas to quickly calculate the percentage of the body that is affected. The percentages change slightly for a child's body.

rule of nines for an adult
9%—head and neck together
9%—each arm
18%—front surfaces of the trunk
18%—rear surfaces of the trunk
1%—genitalia
18%—each leg

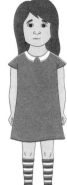

rule of nines for a child
18%—head and neck together
9%—each arm
18%—front surfaces of the trunk
18%—rear surfaces of the trunk
14%—each leg

Another way to estimate burned area

The area of the casualty's palm equals one per cent of the casualty's body surface area. With this information, you can estimate the percentage of the body that is burned.

Critical burns

The burns that are critical, that may be life-threatening or can cause life-long disability or disfigurement include:

- any burn that interferes with breathing, inhalation injuries
- any burn where there is also a serious soft tissue injury or fracture
- any burn where the skin bends, including the hands, elbows, knees, etc.
- all electrical burns, because of internal injuries or cardiac compromise
- most chemical burns
- burns to casualties under two or over fifty years old—they do not tolerate burns well
- burns to casualties who have serious underlying medical conditions including diabetes, seizure disorders, hypertension, respiratory difficulties, or mental illness

Complications of burns

Common complications of burns include:

- shock caused by the loss of blood or blood plasma to the surrounding tissues is the immediate danger
- infection, because burned skin isn't a good barrier to bacteria
- breathing problems if the face or throat is burned, or the casualty has inhaled smoke, fumes or steam
- swelling, as clothing and jewellery will cut off circulation when the area swells

Inhalation injuries

Inhalation injuries occur when the casualty inhales hot steam or hot (superheated) air, smoke or poisonous chemicals.

Signs and symptoms of inhalation injuries include signs of shock:

- dizziness, restlessness, confusion,
- pallor or cyanosis

- abnormal breathing rate or depth

Along with a history of exposure to heat and:

- noisy breathing
- pain during breathing
- burns on the face, especially the mouth and nose
- singed hair on the face or head
- sooty or smoky smell on breath
- sore throat, hoarseness, barking cough, difficulty swallowing

5

The only first aid for someone with suspected inhalation injuries is to get to medical aid quickly. Place a conscious casualty in the semi-sitting position if possible and combat shock.

Recognizing burns

Superficial burn—only the top layer of the skin is damaged

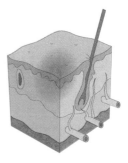

- skin colour is pink to red
- slight swelling
- skin is dry
- tenderness to severe pain in the injured area

Partial Thickness burn—the top two layers of the skin are damaged

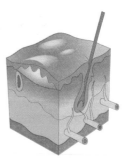

- skin looks raw and is mottled red in colour
- skin is moist and ranges in colour from white to cherry red
- blisters that contain clear fluid
- extreme pain

Full Thickness burn—the full thickness of the skin, including tissues under the skin are damaged

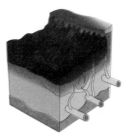

- skin is pearly-white, tan-coloured or charred black

- skin is dry and leathery

- you may see blood vessels and bones under the skin

- little or no pain (nerves are destroyed)

First aid for heat burns

1. Do a scene survey and a primary survey.

2. Cool the burn right away:

   - Immerse it in cool water if possible.

   - If you can't do this, pour cool water on the area or cover it with a clean, wet cloth.

   - Cool the burn until the pain has lessened. This will reduce the temperature of the burned area, and reduce tissue damage, swelling, blistering and relieve the pain.

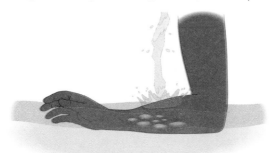

3. Remove jewellery and tight clothing before the injury swells. Don't remove anything that is stuck.

4. When the pain has lessened, loosely cover the burn with a clean, lint-free dressing. If the area is large, use a sheet.

5. Give ongoing casualty care.

Precautions for first aid for burns

- Do not breathe on, cough over or touch the burned area.
- Do not break blisters.
- Do not remove clothing that is stuck to the burned area.
- Do not use butter, lotions*, ointments* or oily dressings on a burn.
- Do not cover a burn with cotton wool or other fluffy material.
- Do not use adhesive dressings.
- Do not cool the casualty too much. Once the area is cooled, take action to keep the casualty warm.

*Sunburn lotions and ointments can be used on minor sunburn.

Burn dressings

A good burn dressing is sterile, lint-free and won't stick to the injury when it is removed. If you don't have something like this, use something clean and lint-free, like a linen sheet. Another type of burn dressing is the "gelled water" burn dressing, e.g. Water-Jel®. These sterile dressings are coated with a jelly-like substance that is mostly water. As such, the dressings are effective in cooling the burn, keeping it clean and providing pain relief. Use these dressings according to the instructions on the package.

First aid for chemical burns

A corrosive chemical will keep burning as long as it is on the skin. The faster you get the chemical off the skin, the less tissue damage there will be.

1. Do a scene survey and a primary survey.

2. Flush the area with large amounts of cool water. Remove contaminated clothing while flushing. If the chemical is a dry powder, quickly brush off any loose chemical with a cloth before flushing.

3. Continue flushing the area with water for 15 to 20 minutes.

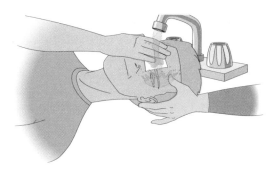

4. When the pain has lessened, loosely cover the burn with a clean, lint-free dressing.

5. Give ongoing casualty care.

5

If you work with chemicals, make sure you know the specific first aid for the chemicals in your workplace. The SDS, safety data sheet, for each chemical contains this information. If you work with chemicals at your place of employment, you are required to be certified in WHMIS.

First aid for electrical burns

Electrical burns can be either flash burns or contact burns.

A **flash burn** results when high voltage electricity arcs (jumps) from the electric source to the casualty. When the electricity arcs, it produces intense heat for a very short time and this heat causes burns, which can be a very deep. The force can throw the casualty as well. Head/spinal injuries, fractures or dislocations may be present.

In a **contact burn**, electricity travels through the body. The body may be burned at both the point where the electricity entered the body and where it exited. There may also be severe tissue damage inside the body, along the path the electricity followed.

An electrical current going through the body can cause breathing to stop and/or the heart to stop. There is also the danger of electrical injury to the first aider.

1. Do a scene survey, then a primary survey. Make sure there is no further danger from electricity; call the power company or other officials to make the scene safe. If high voltages are involved, all you can do is keep others out of the area until the power is shut off.

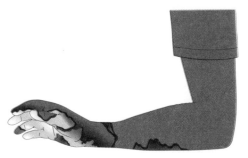

Does it look like the casualty was thrown? If so, suspect a head or spinal injury.

2. Do a secondary survey to locate burns and any fractures, dislocations, etc. Look for both entry and exit burns.

3. Give first aid for the burns by covering them with clean, dry dressings.

4. Give first aid for any fractures or dislocations.

5. Give ongoing casualty care.

When power lines are down

- If there is a possibility of a downed power line or a weakened pole, do not leave your vehicle until you have inspected the surrounding area, looking for downed power lines.

- Stay inside your vehicle if it is touching power lines. Wait for authorities to arrive, then follow their instructions.

- If you suspect or see any downed power lines, don't let anyone enter the area. When you are sure no one will enter the area, notify the power company.

- With high voltages, electricity can travel through the ground, energizing the area around the power lines. If the soles of your feet tingle as you enter an area, you've gone too far—get back.

- Assume all downed power lines are live. A high voltage wire may be unpredictable—it may jump to an object for a better ground. Stay well away from any wires.

- Remember that vehicles, guardrails, metal fences, etc., conduct electricity.

First aid for sunburn

Sunburns can range in severity from those that are mildly uncomfortable to those that are serious because they cover a large area of the body, and can be complicated by heatstroke.

5

For minor sunburn, give first aid as follows:

1. Get out of the sun, and do a scene survey and primary survey.

2. Gently sponge the area with cool water or cover with a wet towel, to relieve the pain. Repeat this step as needed to relieve pain.

3. Pat the skin dry and put on a medicated sunburn ointment if available. Apply the lotion according to directions on the package.

4. Protect burned areas from further exposure to the sun.

5. Don't break any blisters—doing so may promote infection. If large areas of the skin begin to blister, get medical help.

6. If the casualty begins to vomit, or develops a fever, give first aid for heat injuries and get medical help.

First aid for burns from X-rays and nuclear radiation

There is no specific first aid for radiation burns from X-rays or radioactive material. Give first aid following the guidelines for first aid for heat burns. In an environment where there is radioactive material, protect yourself accordingly.

How to put out a fire on your clothes

If your clothing catches fire:

Stop — moving

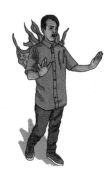

Drop — to the ground

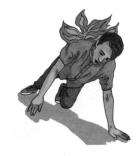

Roll — several times to put flames out

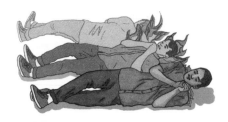

Don't run — this only fans the flames.

How to exit a smoke-filled room

If you can, cover your mouth and nose with a wet cloth

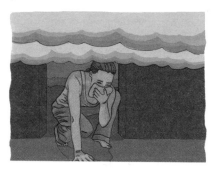

Hot smoke rises—keep your head low as you crawl under the smoke

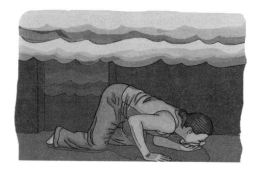

5

Bites and stings

Animal and human bites

Animal and human bites that cause puncture wounds or lacerations may carry contaminated saliva into the body and are dangerous because of the risk of infection. The most common human bites in adults are to the hand. All animal and human bites that break the skin should be seen by a doctor.

Rabies is an acute viral disease of the nervous system that is always fatal if not treated. Rabies should be suspected in domestic animals if they behave in an unusual way, and in all attacks by wild animals (bats, foxes, skunks, raccoons, and more). The rabies virus can be transmitted to anyone who handles a diseased animal or who touches the area of the wound that carries the virus. To be safe, always give first aid for an animal bite as if the animal had rabies, until it is proved otherwise.

Be especially careful when giving first aid to anyone you suspect may have been exposed to rabies and in handling the live or dead animal involved. Wear gloves and/or scrub your hands thoroughly after contact to reduce the risk of infection.

Even if a person has been exposed to a rabid animal, full-blown rabies can be prevented if immunization against the disease is given quickly.

First aid for animal/human bites

1. Perform a scene survey and a primary survey.
2. Examine the wound to see if the skin was broken.
3. If there is bleeding, allow moderate bleeding of the wound— this helps to cleanse the wound.
4. Wash the wound then apply a dressing and bandage.
5. Get medical help.

Snakebite

Rattlesnakes are the only poisonous snakes found in the wild in Canada. Varieties of this snake can be found in parts of British Columbia, Alberta, Saskatchewan and Ontario.

If you are travelling to areas where there are other poisonous snakes, learn the first aid for snakebites in that area.

A rattlesnake's bite leaves one or two puncture holes in the skin. Venom may be injected into the casualty. If it is, the casualty will feel a burning sensation. This is followed by swelling and discoloration, severe pain, weakness, sweating, nausea, vomiting and chills. Breathing may be affected.

5

First aid for snakebite

1. Do a scene survey and primary survey.
2. Place the casualty at rest in a semi-sitting position and keep the affected limb below heart level. By placing the casualty at rest, the venom won't spread as quickly.
3. Flush the bite if possible. Wrap a large roller bandage around the entire length of the bitten extremity, just tight enough that you can get your fingers under the bandage. This is an effective and safe way to slow circulation of the venom.
4. Immobilize the limb.
5. Give ongoing casualty care.

Precautions when dealing with snakes and snakebite

- most snakes will be within 10 metres of the place where the bite took place—be careful

- do not let a snakebite casualty walk if there is any other method of transportation to medical help

- do not give the casualty alcoholic beverages

- do not cut the puncture marks or try to suck poison out with your mouth

- do not apply ice—this could cause more damage

- if the snake is killed, bring it to medical help for identification, but do not touch the snake directly. Avoid the snake's head—a dead snake still may have a bite reflex

Insect bites and stings

An insect bite or sting causes only a painful swelling with redness and itching at the site for most people. But some people are severely allergic to these stings and being stung may cause a life-threatening allergic reaction.

Signs and symptoms of a localized reaction at the site of a bite or sting:

- sudden pain
- swelling
- heat
- redness
- itching

Signs and symptoms of an anaphylactic reaction to a bite or sting:

- general itching, rash
- a bump on the skin that may be white, pink, reddish or blotchy
- generalized swelling—especially of the airway
- weakness, headache
- fever
- breathing difficulties that may be severe
- anxiety, abdominal cramps, vomiting

First aid for an insect bite or sting

1. Do a scene survey, then a primary survey. Are there any signs of an allergic reaction?

2. Looking for a stinger that may still be in the skin. Honey bees leave their stinger and venom sac attached to the skin. Other bees and wasps do not. If it is there, remove it by carefully scraping it and the attached poison sac from the skin.

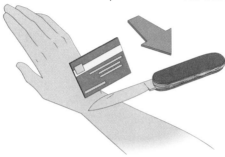

3. For the irritation at the site of the sting, apply rubbing alcohol or a paste of baking soda and water. Ice can also be used. Don't use alcohol near the eyes.

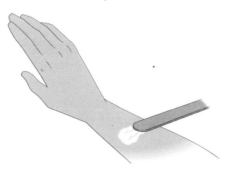

5

Ticks

Ticks are found throughout Canada. They drop from the foliage onto animals and humans, biting through the skin and anchoring themselves to the tissue with barbed mouth parts. A tick will suck the host's (the person or animal) blood for many hours, and may become quite large. Once the tick is done feeding, it detaches itself and drops off.

They sometimes carry diseases that can be transmitted to humans. If one tick is found, check your body and clothing thoroughly for others. Keep the tick for identification by a medical professional.

First aid for bites from ticks

1. Use a tick removal tool to pull out the tick by sliding the tool along the skin and carefully pulling away from the body

2. If you do not have a tick removal tool, use tweezers by grasping the tick close to the skin and carefully pulling at a slow but steady pace. Do not grasp the tick body, as it will pop, spraying the contents

3. If you don't have tweezers, wear gloves or cover your hand with a plastic bag or tissue paper. If the tick is full of blood, wear eye protection.

4. Keep the dislodged tick and bring it to medical help for identification.

5. Clean the area and apply an antiseptic to prevent infection. Ticks can carry various diseases which may cause symptoms several days after exposure. If the tick is found engorged, or if the site of the bite shows any sign of infection or rash (which may look like a halo), get medical help.

Leeches

A leech makes a tiny cut in the skin, which may not be felt at the time, and attaches itself to feed on the blood of a human or animal. Once a leech is attached, trying to pull it off often doesn't work—the leech may tear into smaller parts, making it even harder to remove those parts still attached. This may increase the risk of infection.

First aid for lesions from leeches

1. Detach the leech by first using a fingernail to push the head end of the leech off of the skin. The head end is the smaller, skinnier part of the leech–not the larger end. After the head is released, use a fingernail to push the larger end off.
2. Once the leech is removed, there may be some bleeding due to the anticoagulant produced by the leech. Wash the area with soap and water, and use a baking soda paste or ammonia solution to relieve irritation.
3. If the site of the bite shows any sign of infection, the casualty should get medical help.

Jellyfish

Jellyfish can be found in any body of water, whether salt water or fresh, with different varieties being found in Canada. Jellyfish that have been known to cause death live in tropical climates and have not been located near Canada. All jellyfish sting their prey using nematocysts, which in simple terms are "stingers." These stingers may contain venom which can be harmful, but more commonly cause an unpleasant stinging or burning sensation.

First aid for jellyfish stings

1. Perform a scene survey and a primary survey.
2. Apply as much vinegar as possible to the affected area. Vinegar will stop the stingers from releasing venom.
3. To help relieve pain, bathe the affected part in warm water, as warm as the casualty can tolerate for about 20 minutes.
4. Do not apply cold water. Cold water helps the stingers to continue releasing venom.
5. If signs of infection occur, seek medical help.

5

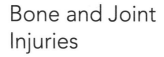

Bone and Joint Injuries

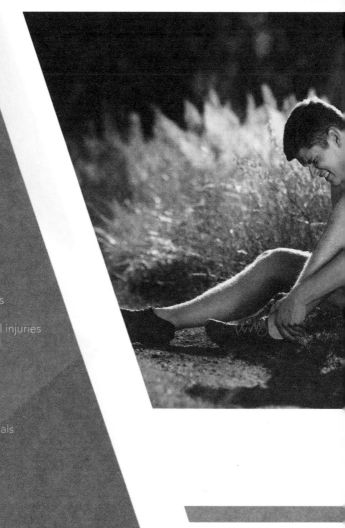

Chapter 6 Bone and joint injuries

Injuries to bones, joints and muscles are common and, although they are usually not life-threatening, they can be painful and debilitating. Appropriate first aid for these injuries can reduce the pain and prevent further injury.

Injuries to bones

A break or crack in a bone is called a fracture. A fracture is either closed or open:

- **a closed fracture** is where the skin over the fracture is not broken

- **an open fracture** is where the skin over the fracture is broken—this could cause serious infection, even if the wound is very small

Closed fracture

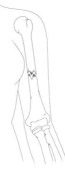

Open fracture

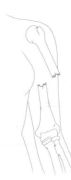

A fracture can be caused by a **direct force** (e.g. a punch or kick), an **indirect force** (e.g. a fall), or by a **twisting force**. Certain **bone diseases**, such as osteoporosis, make bones very brittle and they can break without much force.

One or more of the following **signs and symptoms** will be present when a bone is fractured:

- pain and tenderness—worse when the injury is touched or moved

- loss of function—the casualty cannot use the injured part

- a wound—the bone ends may be sticking out

- deformity—any unnatural shape or unnatural position of a bone or joint

- unnatural movement

- shock—this increases with the severity of the injury

- crepitus—a grating sensation or sound that can often be felt or heard when the broken ends of bone rub together

- swelling and bruising—fluid accumulates in the tissues around the fracture

Injuries to joints

Ligaments connect bones to other bones to form joints, while tendons connect muscles to bones. Ligaments limit the range of movement, support the joint in motion or prevent certain movements altogether. Joints may be injured when the bones and surrounding tissues are forced to move beyond their normal range. When that happens:

- the bones may break, resulting in a fracture

- the ligaments may stretch or tear, resulting in a sprain

- the bone ends may move out of proper position resulting in a dislocation

Sprains

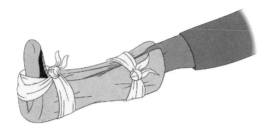

A sprain is an injury to a ligament and can range from a stretched to a completely torn ligament. Be cautious and give first aid as if the injury is serious to avoid further damage and pain. Sprains of the wrist, ankle, knee and shoulder are most common. The **signs and symptoms** of sprains may include:

- pain that may be severe and increase with movement of the joint
- loss of function
- swelling and discoloration

Dislocations

A dislocation is when the bones of a joint are not in proper contact. A force stretches and tears the joint capsule, causing the dislocation. Once this occurs, the bones can put pressure on blood vessels and nerves, causing circulation and sensation impairments below the injury. The most commonly dislocated joints are shoulder, elbow, thumb, fingers, jaw, and knee.

The **signs and symptoms** of a dislocation are similar to those of a fracture, and may include:

- deformity or abnormal appearance, a dislocated shoulder may make the arm look longer
- pain and tenderness aggravated by movement
- loss of normal function; the joint may be "locked" in one position
- swelling of the joint

General first aid for injuries to bones and joints

The aim of first aid for bone and joint injuries is to prevent further tissue damage and to reduce pain.

1. Perform a scene survey and a primary survey.

2. Steady and support any obvious fractures or dislocations found in the primary survey (during the rapid body survey).

3. Do a secondary survey to the extent needed, gently expose the injured area. You may have to cut clothing to do this without moving the injured part. Examine the entire injured area to determine the extent of the injury.

4. Check the circulation below the injury. If circulation is impaired, medical help is needed urgently.

5. Steady and support the injured part and maintain support until medical help takes over, or the injury is immobilized. Protect protruding bones. Do not push the bone ends back in.

   a. If medical help is on the way and will arrive soon, steady and support the injury with your hands until they arrive.

   b. If medical help will be delayed, or if the casualty needs to be transported, immobilize the injury. Consider the following when making your decision:

      • Are there other risks to the casualty? Are there risks to yourself or others?

      • If medical help can get to the scene, how long will it take?

      • Do you have the materials needed to properly immobilize the injury?

      • How long will it take to immobilize the injury compared to how long it will take for medical help to arrive?

7. Apply cold to the injury, as appropriate.

8. Give ongoing casualty care until medical help arrives. Monitor circulation below the injury site.

6

Use RICE for injuries to bones, joints and muscles

Most injuries to bones, joints and muscles benefit from RICE, which stands for:

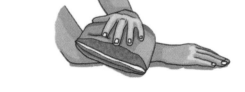

- Rest
- Immobilize
- Cold
- Elevate

Use RICE while waiting for medical help to arrive or while transporting a casualty to medical help. Even the most minor injuries will benefit from RICE.

Rest means stopping the activity that caused the injury and staying off it until a doctor tells the casualty it is OK to continue. For a minor injury, gentle use of the injured part is okay provided the casualty can easily tolerate the pain.

Immobilize means suspecting a fracture whenever there is an injury to an arm or a leg and taking steps to prevent movement of the injured limb. Immobilization may mean using a sling for a shoulder joint injury or a splint to immobilize the joint above and the joint below the injury.

Cold means applying cold to the injury as soon as you can once the injury has been immobilized. The cold narrows the blood vessels, reducing pain, swelling and bruising. Use a commercial cold pack, an improvised ice pack or a cold compress for more about using cold. Apply cold over the entire injured area—15 minutes on, 15 minutes off.

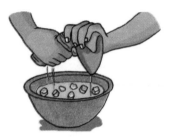

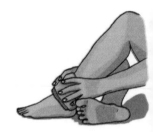

Elevate means raising the injured part if possible. Only elevate if it will not cause more pain or harm to the casualty. Elevation helps to reduce swelling and makes it easier for fluids to drain away from the injury. This in turn, helps reduce swelling (don't elevate a "locked" joint).

Head and spinal injuries

Head injuries include skull fractures, concussion and compression. Such injuries are frequently complicated by unconsciousness. Fractures at the base of the skull often involve injury to the cervical spine. For this reason, when you suspect a head injury, you should also suspect a neck injury.

Injuries associated with the spine/pelvis include fractures, spinal cord damage, and severe bleeding. The bladder is the organ most frequently damaged with pelvic injuries.

A head/spinal injury should be suspected whenever the incident involves a car accident or a fall, from a height of 6 feet or more. It should also be suspected if **signs and symptoms** include:

- fluid from the ears

- headache

- bruising on the head

- casualty complains of pain in the head and neck

- casualty tells you they cannot move or feel

Always suspect head/spinal injury if the casualty is unconscious and the history is unknown.

6

Head injuries

The following **signs and symptoms** indicate a possible fracture of the skull or facial bones, concussion or compression:

- deformed skull
- swollen, bruised or bleeding scalp
- straw-coloured fluid or blood coming from the nose or ear(s)
- bruising around the eyes (black eye) or behind the ears
- nausea, vomiting, especially in children
- confused, dazed, possibly combative
- semi-conscious or unconscious
- stopped breathing or irregular respiration
- very slow pulse rate
- pupils are of unequal size
- pain at the injury site
- weakened or paralyzed arms and/or legs
- pain when swallowing or moving the jaw
- wounds in the mouth
- knocked-out teeth
- shock
- convulsions

An unconscious casualty with a head injury may vomit. Be ready to turn the casualty to the side (as a unit if possible) and clear the airway quickly.

6

Skull fracture

Fractures of the skull may be the result of direct force or an indirect force that is transmitted through the bones. Fractures may occur in the cranium, at the base of the skull, or in the face. Facial fractures include the nose, the bones around the eyes, the upper jaw and the lower jaw. Fractures of the jaw are often complicated by wounds inside the mouth.

First aid for head injury

First aid for fractures of the skull depends on the fracture site and the signs. Whenever there is a skull fracture, a spinal injury should be suspected—give first aid as if there was a neck injury. The head and neck should be immobilized accordingly.

6

1. Perform a scene survey. Assess the mechanism of injury. If you suspect that there may be a head injury tell the casualty not to move and get medical help. Steady and support the head with your hands as soon as possible. Perform a primary survey.

2. If blood or fluid is coming from the ear canal, secure a sterile dressing lightly over the ear, making sure fluids can drain.

3. Protect areas of depression, lumps, bumps, or scalp wounds where an underlying skull fracture is suspected. Avoid pressure on the fracture site.

4. Warn the casualty not to blow their nose if there is blood or fluid coming from it. Do not restrict blood flow. Wipe away any trickling blood to prevent it from entering the mouth, causing breathing difficulties.

5. Give ongoing casualty care until medical help takes over.

First aid for fractures of the facial bones and jaw

1. Perform a scene survey. If you suspect a head injury, tell the casualty not to move and get medical help. Steady and support the head with your hands as soon as possible. Perform a primary survey. Check the airway and make sure there is nothing in the mouth.

2. Remove any knocked-out teeth or loose dentures and maintain drainage for blood and saliva.

3. If there is a suspected head or spinal injury, steady and support the casualty in the position found until medical help takes over.

4. If there is **no** suspected head or spinal injury:

   - place the conscious casualty in a sitting position with head well forward to allow any fluids to drain freely

   - if the casualty cannot sit comfortably, place them in the recovery position

   - place the unconscious breathing casualty in the recovery position.

5. Get medical help and give ongoing casualty care.

If transporting the casualty on a stretcher, ensure good drainage from the mouth and nose so that breathing will not be impaired.

Concussion and compression

Concussion is a temporary disturbance of brain function usually caused by a blow to the head or neck. The casualty may become unconscious but usually for only a few moments. The casualty usually recovers quickly, but there is a chance of serious brain injury. Use both the mechanism of injury and the **signs and symptoms** below to assess for concussion or compression.

- partial or complete loss of consciousness, usually of short duration

- shallow breathing

- nausea and vomiting when regaining consciousness

- casualty says they are (or were) "seeing stars"

- loss of memory of events immediately preceding and following the injury

- severe overall headache (not local scalp pain)

Compression is a condition of excess pressure on some part of the brain. It may be caused by a build-up of fluids inside the skull, or by a depressed skull fracture where the broken bones are putting pressure on the brain. It is very important to monitor a casualty's vital signs and look for other symptoms after a blow to the head.

The **signs and symptoms** of compression are progressive—they usually get worse as time goes on, as more and more pressure is put on the brain.

- loss of consciousness
- decreasing level of consciousness
- nausea and vomiting
- unequal size of pupils
- one or both pupils don't respond to light

6

Helmets

Helmets are designed to protect the wearer from fractures. They are not actually designed to protect against concussion or compression injury. If you see damage to the helmet you should suspect a concussion or compression injury.

Ongoing casualty care for head injury

When a casualty has received a blow to the head or neck that causes decreased consciousness or unconsciousness, immediately suspect a neck injury. Tell the casualty not to move, steady and support the head. Send for medical help and give ongoing casualty care.

A casualty with a concussion may appear to recover quickly, but there is always the threat of serious injury. Tell the casualty to get medical help right away for a full evaluation of the injury.

If the casualty is unconscious and you must leave them alone, place them in the recovery position, carefully supporting the head and neck during any movement. If the casualty is face-up, monitor breathing continuously.

A casualty who shows signs of compression needs to seek medical help immediately.

Spinal injuries

Injury to the spine threatens the spinal cord that runs through it and the nerves that branch out from the cord.

Damage to the spinal cord or nerves can result in complete and permanent loss of feeling and paralysis below the point of injury. In every emergency situation, assess the possibility of a spinal injury. If it exists at all, give first aid for a spinal injury and get medical help as soon as possible.

Use the history of the scene, especially the mechanism of injury, to decide if there is a chance of a spinal injury. If the history of the scene suggests a spinal injury, give first aid for a spinal injury even if the **signs and symptoms** below are not present.

- swelling and/or bruising at the site of the injury

- numbness, tingling or a loss of feeling in the arms and legs on one or both sides of the body

- not able to move arms and/or legs on one or both sides of the body

- pain at the injury site

- signs of shock

Stabilizing a head or spinal injury

The aim of first aid for spinal injuries is to prevent further injury, by preventing movement of the injured area. When moving the casualty is necessary, support them in a way that minimizes movement of the head and spine.

1. As soon as you suspect a head or spinal injury, tell the casualty not to move. Steady and support the casualty's head and neck as soon as you can—show a bystander how to do this:

- Keep elbows on the ground to keep arms steady.
- Firmly hold the head with fingers along the line of the jaw.

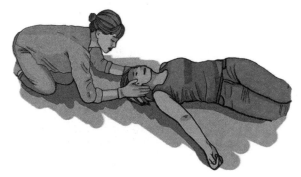

6

Show a second bystander how to steady and support the feet. The head and feet should be continuously supported until either the casualty is fully immobilized or medical help takes over.

Perform a primary survey. If the casualty is unresponsive, check for breathing before opening the airway.

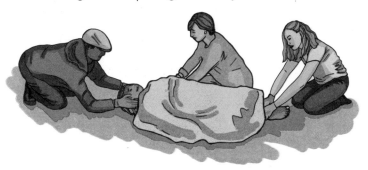

2. Do a secondary survey to the extent needed.

3. If medical help will arrive at the scene, steady and support the casualty in the position found and give ongoing casualty care. Continue to steady and support the head and feet until help arrives.

Pelvic injury

Signs and symptoms of pelvic injury include:

- signs of shock (casualty could be bleeding internally)
- casualty cannot stand or walk
- urge to urinate
- casualty cannot urinate or there is blood in the urine
- sharp pain in the groin and small of the back
- increased pain when moving

Immobilizing a fractured pelvis

Give first aid as you would for a spinal injury. Steady and support the casualty in the position found while waiting for medical help. Stabilize the pelvic area with heavy padding such as blankets on either side.

Chest injury

Signs and symptoms include:

- pain at injury site when casualty moves, coughs or breathes deeply
- shallow breathing
- casualty guards injury
- deformity and discolouration
- may be a wound
- may cough up frothy blood
- may show signs of shock

First aid for chest injury

First aid for injured ribs or breastbone aims to reduce the chance of further injury, to minimize pain and to make breathing easier.

A fracture is very painful and causes shallow breathing. Start ESM.

1. Expose the injured area and look for a wound. If there is a wound, put a dressing on the wound and get medical help quickly.
2. If injuries permit, place the casualty in a semi-sitting position, leaning slightly toward the injured side—this should help breathing. Hand support over the injured area may make breathing easier.
3. Support the arm on the injured side in a St. John tubular sling to restrict movement.
4. Give ongoing casualty care, monitor breathing often. Get medical help.

Flail chest

A flail chest occurs when several ribs in the same area are broken in more than one place. The flail segment moves opposite to the rest of the chest while breathing, which causes pain for the casualty.

Signs and symptoms of a flail chest include:

- paradoxical chest movement—this is the sign that will tell you whether there is a flail chest

- breathing is very painful, and the casualty may support the injured area

- bruising at the injury site

First aid for a flail chest

1. Steady and support the head and neck. Perform a primary survey. If the casualty complains of difficulty breathing and pain in the chest, expose and examine the injury.

2. Support the injured area with your hand—this may make breathing easier. Give first aid for ineffective breathing if needed.

3. Secure the arm to the chest wall with a broad bandage to prevent movement of the arm.

4. Give ongoing casualty care until medical help takes over.

Pneumothorax– a serious complication of a chest injury that requires immediate medical help

The pleural space is the space between the lungs and the chest wall that is filled by the lungs. The lungs expand into this space as the chest cavity changes volume because of the action of the diaphragm and rib cage. But if air gets into the space, the lung on that side won't expand into it, and it will collapse. A pneumothorax occurs when air gets into the pleural space. It is life-threatening because the lungs can collapse and cause the person severe breathing difficulties.

Collarbone/shoulder blade fracture

Signs and symptoms include:

- pain at injury site
- swelling and deformity
- loss of function of the arm on the side of the injury
- casualty holds and protects the arm if they can, and may tilt the head to the injured side

Possible complications

- circulation to the arm below the injury may be impaired or cut off

First aid for a fractured collarbone or shoulder blade

1. Check circulation below the injury. If circulation is impaired, get medical help quickly.

2. Immobilize the arm in the position of most comfort. A St. John tubular sling may work.

- Secure the arm to the chest with a broad bandage to prevent movement of the arm. Pad under the elbow, if necessary, to keep the arm in the most comfortable position. Tie the bandage on the uninjured side—don't tie it so tightly that the arm is pulled out of position. Pad under the knots for comfort.

- Check circulation below the injury. If circulation is impaired, and it was not before, loosen the sling and bandage.

Immobilizing a dislocated joint

Immobilize the limb in the position of most comfort—usually the position found.

To immobilize a dislocated shoulder, if the arm will bend:

- use a St. John tubular sling to transfer the weight of the arm to the other side
- use broad bandages to prevent movement
- pad under the elbow for support

If the arm will not bend:

- support the weight of the arm with a bandage around the neck
- bandage the arm to the body to prevent movement
- pad under the elbow, if necessary, to keep the arm in the most comfortable position
- or the casualty may want to hold the injured arm

The success of the method you use depends on whether it stops the injured limb from moving—which causes pain and could cause further injury. Once the injury is immobilized, apply cold to help reduce pain and swelling providing the casualty can tolerate the added weight.

Monitor circulation below the injury often—check the skin colour and temperature, use a nail bed test and check for a pulse. Compare the injured side with the uninjured side. If circulation becomes impaired after immobilizing the injury, loosen the bandages. If circulation remains impaired, get medical help quickly

6

mmobilizing the upper arm

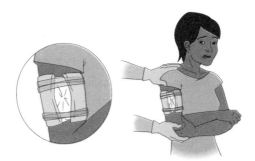

o immobilize an open fracture of the upper arm (humerus):

1. Expose the injury site. Cover the wound with a sterile dressing and check circulation.

2. Pad and bandage the dressings. Pad lengthwise on both sides of the fracture site. Padding should be bulky enough to protect any protruding bone ends. Hold the padding in place with tape then bandage dressings tightly enough to hold padding and dressings in place.

3. An arm sling provides full support for the arm—broad bandages above and below fracture site prevent arm movement. Pad under the elbow as needed to hold the arm in the position of comfort.

6

Immobilizing an injured elbow

The elbow can be severely sprained, fractured or dislocated. Immobilize the injury in the position found, if possible, or in the position of greatest comfort.

1. Expose the injury and look for any open wounds. Check circulation below the injury and compare it with the other side. If circulation is impaired, get medical help quickly.

2. If the elbow is bent so the arm is in front of the chest, immobilize the arm in an arm sling. Leave the sling loose at the elbow. Pad under the elbow, if necessary, to keep the arm in the most comfortable position and use a broad bandage to limit movement.

3. If the elbow will not bend, support the arm at the wrist and use broad bandages and padding to immobilize the arm. Check circulation below the injury and compare it with the other side—if it is impaired, and it wasn't before, adjust the sling and/or bandages.

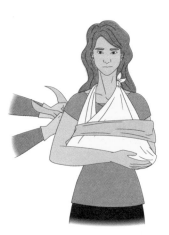
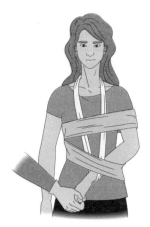

Immobilizing the forearm and wrist

1. Examine the injury and decide the best position for splinting—this is usually in the position found. Have the casualty or a bystander steady and support the injured arm.

2. Measure the splint against the uninjured arm to make sure it is the right size. Pad the splint for comfort and to support the fracture. Position the arm on the splint with as little movement as possible.

3. Once the splint is in position, have the casualty or bystander support it while you secure the splint.

4. Start above the injury and bandage the splint and the arm snugly, but not too tightly. Leave the fingertips visible so you can check circulation below the injury and bandages.

5. Use an arm sling to support the arm and hand, and prevent movement of the elbow with the fingertips exposed so you can check circulation.

6

Immobilizing an injured hand

When you suspect bones in the hand are fractured:

1. Examine the injured hand and decide the best position for splinting—this is usually in the position of function. Have the casualty or a bystander steady and support the injury. If there are open wounds, place non-stick sterile dressings between the fingers to prevent the fingers sticking together.

2. Measure the splint against the uninjured hand and arm to make sure it is the right size.

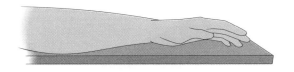

Position the arm on the splint with as little movement as possible.

Using a cushion as a splint

- A cushion or pillow works well because it lets the hand rest in the position of function and it is padded but also firm. It fully supports the wrist and lower arm.

- secure the pillow with 2 broad bandages, making sure there is no pressure on the hand.

- leave fingertips visible to check for circulation.

Using a board

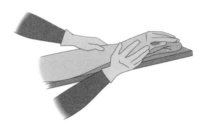

- A board works well because it is rigid, but, you must use padding to keep the hand in the position of function.

- secure the splint with a roller bandage. Leave fingertips visible to check for circulation.

3. Immobilize the arm in an arm sling tied to keep the lower arm and hand supported.

Position of function

The position of function is the position the uninjured hand naturally takes—palm down and fingers slightly curled. This position is safer and more comfortable than trying to flatten the hand against a flat surface.

Immobilizing an injured finger or thumb

Immobilize a fractured or dislocated finger or thumb in the position found.

1. Expose the injury. Check the circulation below the injury.

2. Immobilize the finger or thumb in the position of most comfort, which is usually the position of function. Use a splint, or if a splint is not available, secure the injured finger or thumb to the uninjured finger beside it. Use padding to provide extra support.

3. Put on a St. John tubular sling to keep the injury elevated. Be careful not to put pressure on the injury. Check circulation below the injury.

4. Give ongoing casualty care and get medical help.

Fractured upper leg (femur)

Signs and symptoms
- pain, perhaps severe
- the foot and leg may roll outward
- deformity and shortening of the leg

Possible complications
- there can be internal bleeding, causing severe shock

Immobilizing an injured upper leg (femur)

A common fracture of the upper leg is a break at the neck of the femur. This is often referred to as a broken hip, and most commonly happens to elderly people. In a younger, healthy person, great force is needed to fracture the upper leg—always assess for a head or spinal injury.

Have a bystander steady and support the injured limb.

1. Gather the splinting materials. Measure the splint(s) against the uninjured leg. Put bandages into position. Pad the splints and position them as shown.

2. Tie the bandages from chest to ankle—from the stable end to the unstable end.

3. Give ongoing casualty care. Get medical help.

If you are using a long and a short splint, place bandages at the ankles, calves, knees, above and below the fracture, hips and chest.

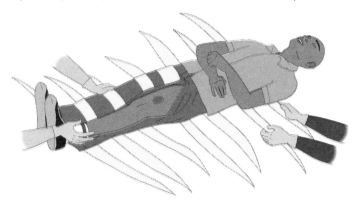

Push bandages under the natural hollows of the body and position as shown above

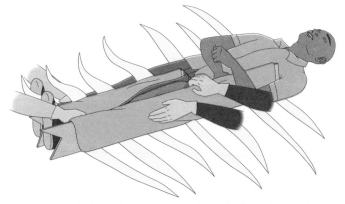

Place splints just below the armpit and just below the groin

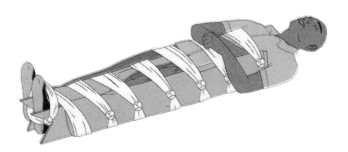

Extend both splints below the foot

Tie off all bandages on the splint

Immobilizing an injured knee

6

Have a bystander steady and support the injured leg. Expose and assess the injury. If the leg is bent, keep it in the position of comfort. Depending on the injury, the casualty may be able to straighten the leg with your help. Don't try to straighten the leg if the pain increases or the leg does not move easily. If the leg won't straighten easily or without increased pain, splint in the position found.

If the leg is straight	**If the leg is bent**
1. Expose and assess the injury	1. Expose and assess the injury

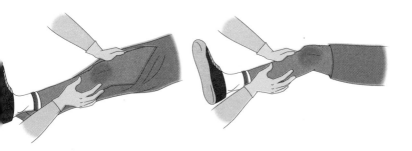

2. Carefully lift the injured leg and position a padded splint

2. Position five broad bandages under the leg—two above the knee and three below

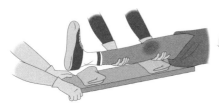

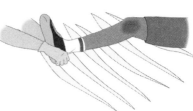

3. Adjust the pads to fit the natural hollows of the leg

3. Position padded splints on the inside and outside of the leg

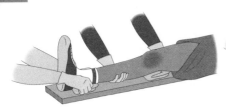

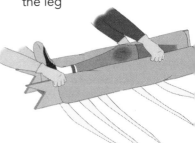

4. Position 2 broad bandages and secure the splint to the leg—use a figure-8 at the ankle

4. Secure the splint with the bandages, keeping the leg in the bent position

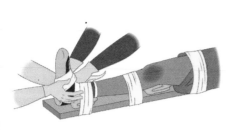

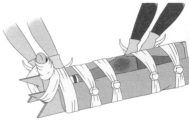

Immobilizing an open fracture of the lower leg (tibia and/or fibula)

When there is an open fracture, give first aid for the wound first and then immobilize the fracture. For the wound, apply a sterile dressing to prevent further contamination. To stop bleeding from the wound, apply pressure around the fracture, but not on it. Apply a dressing with padding on both sides of the fracture site. Secure this with a broad bandage tied tightly enough to put pressure on the padding. Always check circulation before and after dressing a wound of this type.

A fractured lower leg is a common sports injury and open fractures are common. Immobilize a closed fracture the same way but without the dressings and bandages over the wound.

1. Expose the injury. Clothing is removed by cutting to minimize movement of the injured leg.

6

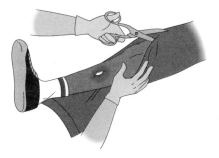

A fracture is "open" when the skin is broken—the bone may stick out

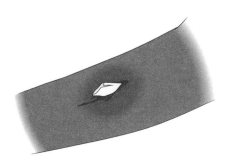

2. Show a bystander how to steady and support the leg. Check the circulation below the injury. Give first aid for the open fracture wound. Leave the shoe on unless there is a wound to be examined.

Cover the wound with a sterile dressing.

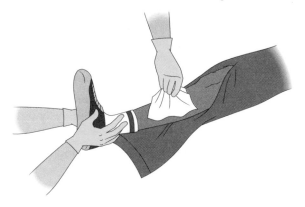

The dressing should extend well beyond the edges of the wound. Put bulky padding lengthwise on both sides of the fracture, over the dressing, to protect the bone end and tape the padding in place.

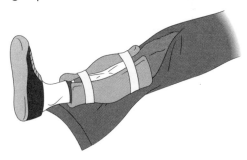

Tie a bandage over the padding and dressing tightly enough to put pressure on the padding, but not tight enough to cut off circulation—check circulation below the injury once the bandage is tied. Make sure there is no pressure on the bone ends.

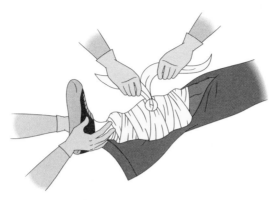

3. Immobilize the lower leg. Position the bandages and splints. Use splints long enough to extend from the groin to below the foot. The bystander doesn't let go of the leg until the first aider tells them to, which is after the last bandage is tied. Tie all knots on the splint for comfort.Position broad bandages to be tied at the thigh, knee, above and below the fracture and at

6

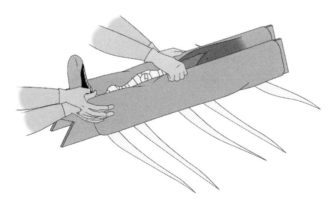

the ankle.

4. Tie the bandages starting at the thigh (the stable end) and working down. The bandage at the ankles is tied as a figure-8.

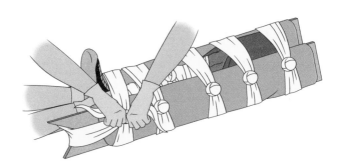

6

5. Check the circulation below the injury; give ongoing casualty care. Get medical help.

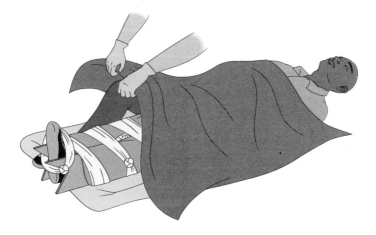

If you don't have splints ...

Use the uninjured leg as an anatomical splint by tying the legs together.

Position padding between the legs (rolled-up blanket).

Position and tie broad bandages at the thighs, knees, above the injury, below the injury and at the ankles. Tie a figure-8 at the ankles.

Tie knots on padding for comfort.

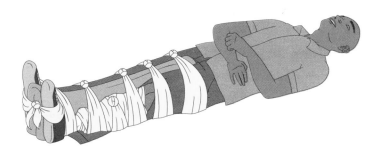

Immobilizing an injured ankle

The ankle should be immobilized whenever you suspect a sprain or a fracture. If the injury doesn't seem serious, or if the journey to medical help will be smooth, use a blanket splint or pillow splint to immobilize the ankle:

1. Check circulation below the injury.

2. Loosen footwear and immobilize the ankle with a pillow or rolled-up blanket and two broad bandages. Make sure the splint extends beyond the ankle.

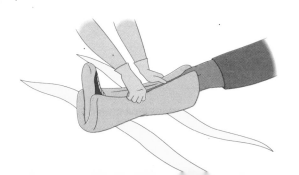

Secure the pillow with two broad bandages—use a figure8 at the ankle.

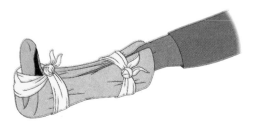

3. Check circulation below the injury. Give ongoing casualty care and get medical help.

Immobilizing an injured foot or toe

6

1. Check circulation below the injury.

2. Immobilize the ankle using a double figure–8.
   Untie shoe laces and tie the first figure–8 beginning at the sole of the foot and tying toward the leg.

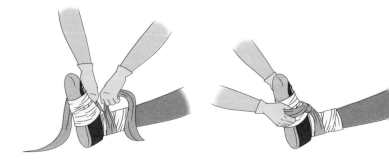

Tie the second figure–8 by wrapping the ends around the leg, crossing in front of the ankle and tying off on the sole of the foot. Tie off at the sole.

Immobilize a fractured toe by taping it to the uninjured toe beside it.

Keep checking circulation, the injured area may swell.

Strains

When a muscle or tendon is moved beyond its normal range, this results in a strain, which is a stretch or tear injury.

The **signs and symptoms** of a strain often show up many hours after the injury.

- sudden sharp pain in the strained muscle
- swelling of the muscles causing severe cramps
- bruising and muscle stiffness
- casualty may not be able to use the affected body part (loss of function)

First aid for strains

1. Perform a scene survey and a primary survey. Have the casualty stop the activity that caused the injury.

2. Place the casualty in a position of comfort and assess the injury. If there is loss of function, immobilize the injury as for a fracture. Manage with RICE.

3. Give ongoing casualty care. Get medical help. Position the casualty on the back with knees raised, or any preferable comfortable position at rest.

6

Splinting materials

A splint is any material used to prevent fractured bones from moving unnecessarily.

A good splint is. . .

- rigid enough to support the injured limb
- well-padded for support and comfort
- long enough, which means:

  ▶ for a fracture between 2 joints, it extends beyond the joints above and below the fracture

  ▶ for an injured joint, it's long enough for the limb to be secured so the joint can't move

6

Commercial splints

There are many commercial splints available. You may have access to one of these if the incident happened at a workplace, sporting event, etc. It is important to be familiar with the splints before use. Always follow the manufacturer's directions.

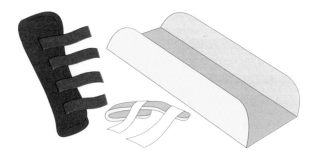

Improvised splints

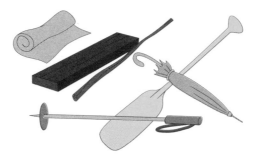

A splint can be improvised from any material, as long as it works to immobilize the injury.

The casualty's own body can be used as a splint; one leg can be splinted to the other for example. This is called an "anatomical" splint.

Other materials needed for splinting

To put the splint on, you will need materials for padding and bandages.

Padding does two things:

- it fills in the natural hollows between the body and the splint, ensuring the injured limb is properly supported

- it makes the splint more comfortable

Always pad between a splint and the injured limb, and between two body parts to be bandaged together.

When using bandages:

- make sure they are wide enough to provide firm support without discomfort

- pass them under the natural hollows of the body—go under the knee, the small of the back, the hollow behind the ankles

- tie them tightly enough to prevent movement, but not so tight they cut off circulation. Check circulation every 15 minutes below any bandages you've tied

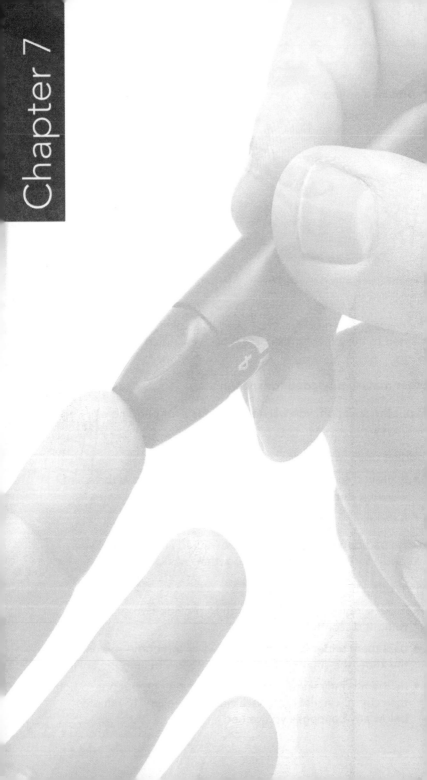

Other First Aid Emergencies

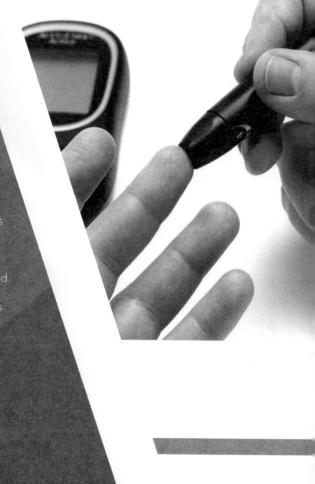

Chapter 7 Other first aid emergencies

Diabetes

Diabetes is a condition in which there is either not enough insulin in the blood or there is enough insulin but the cells cannot use the insulin properly. Insulin is a hormone produced in the pancreas that regulates the amount of glucose in the blood. With diabetes, sugar builds up in the blood and the cells don't get the energy they need or the blood sugar levels can go abnormally low.

A person with diabetes may take medication by mouth or injection, and carefully controls what they eat (the source of energy) and their level of exercise (the use of energy). A diabetic emergency occurs when there is too much or too little insulin in the blood.

- **hypoglycemia**—not enough sugar, too much insulin
- **hyperglycemia**—too much sugar, not enough insulin

Causes, signs and symptoms of diabetic emergencies		
	hypoglycemia (needs sugar)	**Hyperglycemia (needs insulin)**
time to develop	develops very quickly	develops over hours or days
possible cause	– took too much insulin or oral diabetes medication – not eaten enough, or vomited – more exercise than usual	– did not take enough insulin – eating too much food – less exercise than usual – casualty has an ongoing illness and needs more insulin
pulse/breathing	strong and rapid/shallow	weak and rapid/deep and sighing
skin condition	sweaty, pale and cold	flushed, dry and warm

7

level of consciousness	faintness to unconscious	drowsy, becoming unconscious
other signs and symptoms	– headache – confused, irritable and aggressive – trembling, staggering – difficulty speaking	– thirsty, then nausea and vomiting – frequent urination – breath has a nail polish (acetone) like odour

First aid for diabetic emergencies

The aim of first aid in a diabetic emergency is to keep the casualty's condition from getting worse while you get medical help.

1. Perform a scene survey, then do a primary survey.

2. If the casualty is conscious, ask what is wrong.

- A diabetic casualty may have glucose tablets for treating hypoglycemia. Help them take their tablets if they are able to respond and swallow; repeat if symptoms persist after 10 minutes.

- If glucose tablets are not available, use other types of dietary sugars (in order of preference): glucose candy (e.g. Mentos), sucrose candy (e.g. Skittles), jelly beans, orange juice, fructose (e.g. fruit leather), and whole milk.

3. Give ongoing casualty care. Send for medical help

Seizures and convulsions

A **seizure** is caused by abnormal electrical activity in the brain. In a **partial seizure**, only part of the brain is affected. The person may experience a tingling or twitching in one area of the body. In a **generalized seizure**, the whole brain is affected and the person loses consciousness and may have convulsions. A **convulsion** is an abnormal muscle contraction, or series of muscle contractions, that the person cannot control.

Epilepsy is a disorder of the nervous system characterized by seizures. Many people with seizure disorders like epilepsy take medication to control the condition. Other causes of seizures include:

7

- head or brain injury
- stroke
- brain infection
- drug overdose
- a high fever in infants and children

With epilepsy, the person may know that a seizure is about to occur because of a brief sensation they experience, called an **aura**. The aura, which may be a hallucinated sound, smell, or a feeling of movement in the body, is often felt just before a seizure.

A typical generalized seizure has **two phases:**

The **"tonic" phase** involves a sudden loss of consciousness causing the person to fall. The person's body becomes rigid for up to a minute during which the face and neck may turn bluish.

In the **"clonic" phase**, convulsions occur, breathing is noisy, frothy saliva may appear around the mouth and the teeth may grind.

A major seizure can come on very suddenly, but seldom lasts longer than a few minutes.

When the seizure is over, the muscles gradually relax and the person regains consciousness. After the seizure, the person may not remember what happened. They may appear dazed and confused, and feel exhausted and sleepy.

Signs and symptoms of a generalized seizure

- a sudden cry, stiffening of the body and loss of consciousness causing the person to fall
- noisy breathing and frothy saliva at the mouth
- the body jerks
- breathing may stop or be irregular for a minute—the casualty may turn blue
- loss of bladder and bowel control

First aid for a seizure or convulsion

First aid for a seizure aims to protect the casualty from injury during convulsions and to keep the airway open while the casualty is unconscious.

1. Perform a scene survey. Make the area safe—clear away objects that could cause injury. Clear onlookers away to ensure the casualty's privacy.

During convulsions:

- Do not restrict the casualty's movements. Protect them from injury.

- Carefully loosen tight clothing, especially around the neck.

- Place something soft under the head.

- Do not try to put anything in the mouth, between the teeth or to hold the tongue. Perform a primary survey after convulsions are finished.

2. Place the unconscious casualty into the recovery position and clear any fluids from the mouth or nose.

3. Do a secondary survey to see if the casualty was injured during the seizure; give first aid for any injuries.

4. Give ongoing casualty care, monitoring breathing, keeping the casualty warm and allowing them to rest.

- don't give the casualty any liquids during or immediately after a seizure

Call for medical help if:

- the casualty is unconscious for more than five minutes, or has a second major seizure within a few minutes

- this is the person's first seizure or the cause of the seizure is unknown (ask the casualty when they regain consciousness)

7

First aid for a fever emergency in an infant or child

A rapid rise in temperature to 40°C (104°F) or higher can cause convulsions in infants and children. A fever emergency is when the temperature, taken in the armpit (or follow manufacture directions on digital thermometer), is:

- 38o C (100.5o F) or higher for an infant
- 40o C (104o F) or higher for a child

1. Perform a scene survey, then do a primary survey.

2. Call a doctor immediately and follow their advice. If the doctor can't be reached give acetaminophen (e.g. Tempra® or Tylenol®) or children's ibuprofen (not ASA) according to the directions on the label. This should bring down the child's temperature.

3. Encourage the fully conscious child to drink clear fluids.

4. If the temperature doesn't go down, sponge the child with lukewarm water for about 20 minutes, their temperature will go down quickly if the wet skin is exposed to air.

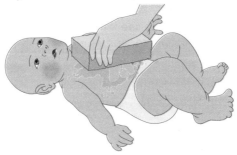

5. Dry and dress the child in comfortable but not overly warm clothing. Monitor the child's temperature and repeat steps 3 to 5, as necessary, until medical help is reached.

6. If the child has a convulsion:

- do not restrain the child, but protect them from injury
- loosen constrictive clothing

7. When the convulsions stop, perform a primary survey.

8. Give ongoing care; place the child into the best recovery position for their age.

Do not give ASA (e.g. Aspirin®) to children or adolescents because it may cause Reye's syndrome, a life-threatening condition.

Do not use cold water when sponging the child—this may cause more serious problems. Only use lukewarm water.

Cold-related injuries

Core body temperature drops when the body loses more heat than it produces. In an outdoor emergency, heat loss by conduction and convection (wet and wind) are often the main contributors to hypothermia.

The body has a number of ways to minimize heat loss and keep the body core warm. One of the first things the body does when it is losing heat is start shivering. If the body keeps getting colder, the blood vessels in the arms, legs and at the skin surface get smaller. This keeps the blood in the core, where it is warmest.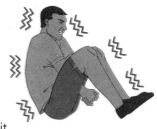

If heat loss continues, the body processes get slower, including thinking, muscular action and the senses. Shivering will become uncontrollable and then will slow down and eventually stop. The muscles get stiff and movements become jerky. Thinking is confused, speech difficult and the senses dulled. The heart and breathing rates slow down and the person eventually loses consciousness. At this point, the condition is very serious. The heartbeat becomes unsteady and faint, and finally the heart stops.

When the heart stops beating, the person is considered dead. However, when body tissues are cold, they aren't damaged as easily by a lack of oxygen. For this reason, there is often a chance of resuscitating a hypothermic person who doesn't show any signs of life. This means that as long as you aren't putting yourself or others at risk, you should continue your rescue efforts to get a hypothermic casualty to medical help.

7

How the body loses heat—examples and prevention			
Heat loss	Explanation	Example	Sample Prevention
1. Radiation	Heat radiates from the body into the air around it.	A lot of heat radiates from the skin.	Wear warm clothes.
2. Breathing	Cold air is inhaled, warmed by the body and exhaled, causing heat loss.	The steam you see when you exhale on a cold day is cold air that your body has just warmed, and lost heat in doing so.	Wear a parka with a "tunnel" hood or "ski-tube"—the air you breath will be warmer than the outside air.
3. Evaporation	Body heat is used to evaporate liquid on the skin.	Sweating is how your body tries to keep cool on a hot day.	Keep your skin as dry as possible.
4. Conduction	Heat moves directly from the body to a cold object that the body is touching	Sitting on the cold ground or wearing wet clothing—your heat moves from you into the ground or wet clothing.	Don't get wet. Wear fabric next to your skin that moves the wet away (e.g. polypropylene)
5. Convection (wind chill)	The thin layer of warm air around the body is replaced by cooler air, which the body must now heat.	The wind blows through openings in your clothing and blows the warm air against your skin away.	Wear windproof clothing with snug cuffs and collars to keep the wind out.

Hypothermia

The normal temperature of the body's core is 37° C (98.6° F). If the body core temperature drops more than two degrees, the body's tissues cannot function properly. This state of generalized cooling is called hypothermia. Hypothermia, often referred to as exposure, kills many Canadians each year—but it is a condition that can be detected and corrected by a first aider if recognized early.

Anyone can become hypothermic, but the following groups are especially prone:

- **elderly people**, because they often have poor circulation, less ability to sense the cold, and may be on medication that promotes heat loss

- **babies** have less ability to recover from mild and moderate hypothermia because they lose heat more quickly and their bodies don't control body heat as well

- people who are already **weakened due to illness**, injury, lack of food, fatigue or through the use of alcohol or drugs

- **teenagers**, because they often underdress for the weather conditions

Signs of hypothermia			
Sign	Mild	Moderate	Severe
pulse	normal	slow and weak	weak, irregular or absent
breathing	normal	slow and shallow	slow or absent
appearance	shivering, slurred speech	shivering violently , clumsy, stumbling, pupils dilated, skin bluish	shivering has stopped
mental state	conscious but withdrawn or disinterested	confused, sleepy irrational	unconscious

7

Signs of hypothermia

There are three stages of hypothermia: **mild, moderate and severe**, but it may be hard to tell exactly when one stage ends and another begins. Body temperatures are not listed here because the first aider has no practical way to take the temperature of the body's core.

The key to successful first aid for hypothermia is recognizing the casualty's condition as soon as possible, and preventing hypothermia from getting worse. Hypothermia is the obvious thing to look for on a cold winter day, but it is less obvious when the temperature is above zero. Be on the lookout for hypothermia whenever the temperature is below 20° C, the weather is windy, wet or both, or the casualty is in one of the groups at risk for hypothermia. Don't forget yourself—as soon as you begin to shiver, think "I've got to prevent further heat loss." If you don't, hypothermia will soon affect your mind, and you won't be able to think clearly enough to take the right actions.

First aid for hypothermia

First aid for hypothermia aims to prevent further heat loss and get medical help.

1. Perform a scene survey and a primary survey.

2. Take measures to prevent further heat loss:

- Move the casualty out of the cold environment. If you cannot move indoors, protect the casualty from the wind.

- Cover exposed skin with suitable clothing or covers.

- If you are in a shelter and have a dry change of clothes, gently replace wet clothes with dry ones. If you are not sheltered, put the dry clothes over the wet clothes.

- If you don't have dry clothes, press as much water out of the wet clothes as possible and wrap the casualty with something windproof.

- Insulate the casualty from cold objects—have them sit on a rolled-up jacket or lie on a blanket.

3. Give the casualty warm sweet drinks if they are conscious.

4. Give ongoing casualty care, get medical help.

Immersion hypothermia

Immersion hypothermia refers to hypothermia caused by being in cold water. A person loses heat 25-30 times faster in water than in air of the same temperature. Immersion hypothermia can happen very quickly if a person falls into cold water. Suspect hypothermia whenever someone falls into water by mistake even in the summer. Immersion hypothermia can also happen more slowly, for instance while swimming or scuba diving in a lake. In these cases, hypothermia creeps up on the casualty, and may not be suspected right away.

Do the following when a hypothermic casualty is in the water:

- Tell the casualty not to take off any clothing—clothing helps keep heat in.

- Tell the casualty to move as little as possible—moving around causes more heat loss (by convection).

When taking a casualty out of the water, keep them in a horizontal position, and handle them as gently as possible. Give first aid for hypothermia to prevent further heat loss, and get medical help.

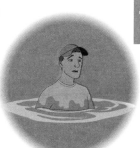

If you are the casualty, use the "heat escape lessening position" (HELP) to preserve body heat.

Rewarming a casualty

There are two types of rewarming: **passive rewarming** and **active rewarming**. Passive rewarming means preventing further heat loss and letting the casualty's body rewarm itself; this usually works well for mild and moderate hypothermia. Active rewarming means adding heat to the casualty's body to warm it up. Active rewarming can cause complications and should only be done at a hospital—but active rewarming is what a casualty in severe hypothermia needs. This is why in severe hypothermia, the first aid is to prevent further heat loss and get medical help.

In **mild** hypothermia, you can give the fully conscious casualty something warm and sweet to drink. The sweetened drink will provide energy to the muscles and help the body to continue shivering.

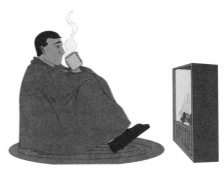

Don't give a casualty in **moderate** hypothermia anything to drink. Their muscles for swallowing may not work well and they could choke, you should actively rewarm the casualty only if you are far from medical aid. Do this by placing the casualty near a heat source and placing containers of warm, but not hot, water in contact with the skin (neck, armpits, groin). Prevent further heat loss and get medical help as soon as possible.

7

Cautions in first aid for hypothermia

- Handle the casualty very gently and keep them horizontal if possible. Cold affects the electrical impulses that make the heartbeat. As a result, the hypothermic casualty's heart beat is very delicate. The heart can stop with rough handling of the casualty.

- Don't give the casualty any alcohol, coffee, or other drinks with caffeine, or let them smoke —these can increase heat loss.

- Don't rub the casualty's body to improve circulation—this will cause cold blood to flow back to the body core and cool the body further.

Frostbite

Frostbite refers to the freezing of tissues when exposed to temperatures below zero. It is a progressive injury with two stages: **superficial frostbite** and **deep frostbite**.

Stages of frostbite and their signs and symptoms

Stage	Description	Signs & symptoms
Superficial frostbite	The full thickness of the skin is frozen. 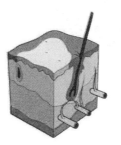	– white, waxy-looking skin – skin is firm to touch, but tissue underneath is soft – may feel pain at first, followed by numbness
Deep frostbite	The skin and the tissues underneath the skin are frozen, sometimes to the bone. A serious condition, often involving an entire hand or foot. 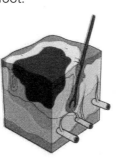	– white, waxy-looking skin that turns greyish-blue as frostbite progresses – skin feels cold and hard – there is no feeling in the area

7

First aid for superficial frostbite

1. Gradually rewarm the frostbitten part with body heat.

- Cover frostbitten toes, ears, etc. with warm hands.

- Warm up frostbitten fingers by placing them in a warm area of the body like the armpit.

2. Take measures to prevent these areas from freezing again—either stop the activity or dress more appropriately.

First aid for deep frostbite

Deep frostbite needs medical help as soon as possible.

1. Prevent further heat loss from the frozen part and the rest of the body. Handle the frozen tissue gently to prevent tissue damage

2. Get medical help. If the feet or legs are frozen, transport using a rescue carry or stretcher if possible.

3. If medical help is not available, you are in a safe, warm place and there is no danger of the part refreezing, then thaw the frozen part:

- Gently remove the clothing from the affected part.

- Find a container that is large enough to hold the entire frozen part and fill this with water that feels warm when you put your elbow in it (about 40° C).

- Remove any jewellery and put the whole frozen part in the water. Keep adding warm water to keep the water in the container at a constant temperature.

- Keep the part in the water until it is pink or does not improve any more—this can take up to 40 minutes, and may be painful.

- Gently dry the affected part. Put sterile dressings over wounds and between fingers or toes.

- Keep the part elevated and warm. Do not break any blisters that form.

4. Give ongoing casualty care.

A deeply frostbitten extremity will be very painful as it defrosts. There will be swelling and perhaps tissue loss. For that reason it is best done at a medical facility. If the casualty must walk out or be transported, do not thaw the frozen part—there will be less tissue damage and pain if the part is left frozen. Make sure the rest of the body is well protected from the cold and the casualty has plenty of food and water during the journey to safety.

Frozen state

When the temperature is below zero, it is possible to discover someone who is completely frozen—this is a frozen state. Recognize a frozen state when:

- the casualty is found in a cold location and is unresponsive
- the joints of the jaw and neck are rigid when you try to open the airway
- the skin and deeper tissues are cold and cannot be depressed
- the entire body moves as a solid unit

7

If the casualty is in a frozen state, do not attempt first aid for the ABCs. Transport the casualty to medical help if this doesn't pose a risk to the rescuers. Otherwise, get yourself to safety and advise the police of the location of the frozen person.

Cautions in first aid for frostbite

- Do not rub the area—the tiny ice crystals in the tissues may cause more tissue damage.
- Do not rub snow on the area—this may cause further freezing and tissue damage from the rubbing.
- Do not apply direct heat; this may rewarm the area too quickly.

Heat related injuries

Prolonged exposure to extreme heat or heavy exertion in a hot environment can cause heat illnesses.

Heat cramps

Heat cramps are painful muscle cramps, usually in the legs and abdomen, caused by losing too much water and electrolytes through sweating. Heat cramps are usually caused by heavy exercise or physical work in a hot environment. The casualty will complain of cramps and show signs of excessive sweating, though in a dry environment, the casualty may not seem to be sweating because the sweat evaporates so quickly.

First aid for heat cramps

1. Place the casualty at rest in a cool place.
2. Give the conscious casualty water or drinks with electrolytes and carbohydrates, as much as they want.

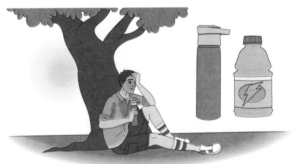

3. If the cramps don't go away, get medical help.

Heat exhaustion

Heat exhaustion is more serious than heat cramps. The casualty has lost a lot of fluids through sweating. Circulation is affected as the blood flows away from the major organs and pools in the blood vessels just below the skin.

Signs and symptoms of heat exhaustion

- excessive sweating and dilated pupils
- casualty may complain of dizziness, blurred vision, headache or cramps
- signs of shock, including: cold, clammy skin; weak, rapid pulse; rapid, shallow breathing; vomiting and unconsciousness

First aid for heat exhaustion

First aid for heat exhaustion combines the first aid for heat cramps with the first aid for shock.

1. If the casualty is **conscious**:

- give the conscious casualty water or drinks with electrolytes and carbohydrates; if the casualty vomits, don't give anything by mouth and get medical help right away
- place them at rest on their back in a cool place
- remove excessive clothing and loosen tight clothing at the neck and waist

2. If the casualty is **unconscious**:

- place them in the recovery position
- get medical help right away

3. Give ongoing casualty care until medical help takes over.

Heatstroke (hyperthermia or sunstroke)

Heatstroke is a life-threatening condition where the body's temperature rises far above normal. It is caused by prolonged exposure in a hot, humid, and perhaps poorly ventilated environment. In classic heatstroke, the body's temperature control mechanism fails; sweating stops and the body temperature rises rapidly. In exertional heatstroke, the body temperature rises rapidly due to heavy physical exertion in high humidity and temperature, even though sweating continues. Elderly people and those in poor health are more likely to suffer from heatstroke. Without immediate first aid heatstroke can result in permanent brain damage or death.

7

Signs and symptoms of heatstroke

- body temperature rapidly rises to 40°C or higher—the casualty is hot to the touch

- the pulse is rapid and full but gets weaker in later stages

- breathing is noisy

- skin is flushed, hot and dry in classic heatstroke, and flushed, hot and sweaty in exertional heatstroke

- casualty is restless and may complain of headache, fatigue, dizziness and nausea

- vomiting, convulsions, unconsciousness may occur

You can tell the difference between heat exhaustion and heatstroke by the condition of the skin. In heat exhaustion, the skin is moist and cold. In heatstroke, the skin is hot, flushed and may be dry or wet.

First aid for heatstroke

1. Perform a scene survey and a primary survey. Lowering body temperature is the most urgent first aid for heatstroke.

- Move the casualty to a cool, shaded place.

- Cool the casualty—remove outer clothing and immerse the casualty in cool water up to the chin—watch them closely. If this is not possible:

- Cover them with wet sheets and fan the sheets to increase cooling.

- Sponge the casualty with cool water, or

- Place cold packs in the armpits, neck and groin areas.

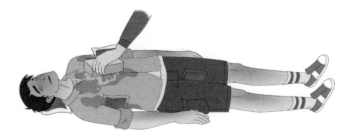

2. When their body feels cool to touch, cover with a dry sheet. Put the conscious casualty into the shock position and the unconscious casualty into the recovery position. If their temperature begins to rise again, repeat the cooling process.

3. Give ongoing casualty care until handover to medical help.

Lightning injuries

Electrical storms occur throughout most of Canada. Although the chance of being struck by lightning is very low, there are many injuries and deaths each year from lightning strikes.

Give first aid at the scene of a lightning strike as you would any other emergency scene, keeping the following in mind:

- a person struck by lightning does not hold an electrical charge, you can touch the casualty without fear of electric shock

- the casualty has probably been thrown—suspect a head or spinal injury

- lightning does strike the same place twice—assess the risk of another strike, and move to a safer location if needed

- if more than one person is injured, the principles of multiple casualty management are reversed—give first aid to unresponsive non-breathing casualties first since the casualties still breathing are on the road to recovery

- advise all casualties of a lightning strike to seek medical help to ensure a full evaluation of any injuries

7

Poisoning

A poison is any substance that can cause illness or death when absorbed by the body. There are poisonous substances all around us. Poisonous consumer products have poison symbols on their labels, but there are many other poisonous substances that don't carry warnings. Examples include alcohol, some common household plants, contaminated food, and medications when not taken as prescribed. Many substances that are not harmful in small amounts may be poisonous in large amounts.

Poisons are classified according to how they enter the body:

- **swallowed poisons**—through the mouth
- **inhaled poisons**—through the lungs
- **absorbed poisons**—through the skin and mucous membranes
- **injected poisons**—through a hollow needle or needle-like device (e.g. a snake's fangs)

An important part of the first aid for poisoning is telephoning your local or provincial **poison information centre** for advice on what to do. Before calling, the first aider must quickly gather as much information about the incident as possible. Use the history of the scene and the signs and symptoms of the casualty to gather the information you'll need to answer the questions asked by the poison information centre.

History of the scene

You need to know four basic facts to give appropriate first aid for poisoning:

- what poison was taken—container labels should identify the poison; otherwise, save vomit and give it to medical help for analysis. What was taken will often tell you -
- how the poison entered the body—first aid may differ for poisons taken by mouth, absorbed through the skin, injected into the blood or breathed into the lungs
- how much poison was taken—estimate the quantity that may have been taken based on what you see or are told— the number of pills originally in the container, the amount

of chemical in the bottle, etc. Estimate the size/age of the casualty, the smaller the person the more dangerous the dosage.

- when the poison was taken—the length of time the poison has been in the body will help determine the first aid and medical care needed

Signs and symptoms of poisoning

If the history does not reveal what poison was taken, or by what means it was taken, signs and symptoms may be helpful in answering these questions. All poisons may affect consciousness, breathing and pulse. Other signs and symptoms may vary depending on how the poison was taken. Poisons that have been:

- swallowed usually cause nausea, abdominal cramps, diarrhea and vomiting. They may discolour the lips, cause burns in or around the mouth or leave an odour on the breath

- absorbed through the skin may cause a reddening of the skin, blisters, swelling and burns

- injected through the skin usually irritate the point of entry

- inhaled may cause coughing, chest pain and difficulty breathing

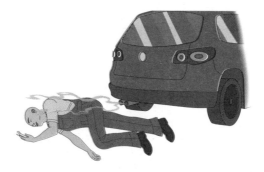

Note that some poisonous gases (i.e. carbon monoxide) are colourless and odourless. They are not to be easily detectable. Exercise extra caution if inhaled poisoning is suspected.

General first aid for poisoning

1. Perform a scene survey. Do a primary survey. Gather any information about the suspected poison.

2. If the casualty is responsive, call the poison information centre in your region and follow their advice.

3. If the casualty is unresponsive or having a seizure, call for medical help.

4. If the casualty is unresponsive but breathing, place in the recovery position.

5. Give ongoing casualty care until medical help takes over.

First aid for swallowed poisons

1. Perform a scene survey and a primary survey.

2. Do not dilute a poison that has been swallowed (do not give fluids) unless told to do so by the Poison Information Centre.

3. If the casualty is conscious, wipe poisonous or corrosive residue from the casualty's face and rinse or wipe out the mouth.

4. Never induce vomiting except on the advice of the Poison Information Centre—many poisons will cause more damage when vomited.

First aid for inhaled poisons

1. Perform a scene survey and a primary survey. Assess hazards with particular attention to the possible presence of a poisonous gas or vapour. Ensure your safety; it may be best to wait for professional rescuers.

2. Move the person to fresh air and away from the source of the poison.

3. If breathing is not present begin CPR. If the poison could affect you while giving first aid, use a face mask or shield with a one-way valve.

4. If the casualty vomits, keep the airway open by clearing out the mouth and putting the casualty into the recovery position.

7

5. If the casualty goes into convulsions, prevent them from injuring themself.

6. Give ongoing casualty care. Get medical help.

First aid for absorbed poisons

Most poisons absorbed by the skin cause irritation at the place of contact, but don't affect the rest of the body. The irritation, called contact dermatitis, includes redness, itching and blisters. Some chemicals, however, do affect the rest of the body when absorbed by the skin, and these can cause life-threatening emergencies.

1. Perform a scene survey and a primary survey.

2. Flush the affected area with large amounts of cool water; if the poisonous substance is a powder, brush off excessive amounts with a dry cloth before flushing.

3. Remove any clothing that has been in contact with the poison. Don't touch the clothing until it has been thoroughly washed.

4. Wash the affected skin thoroughly with soap and water.

5. Give ongoing casualty care until medical help takes over.

First aid for injected poisons

Follow the general first aid for poisoning. Injected poisons should be contained near the injection site. Delay the circulation of the poison throughout the body by placing the casualty at rest and keeping the affected limb below heart level.

If you have been pricked with a needle with possible transmissible disease contamination, then the site of the needle-stick injury should be vigorously scrubbed with Iodine or similar disinfectant. Get medical attention.

Emergency childbirth and miscarriage

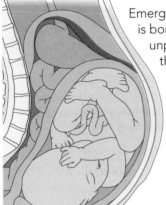

Emergency childbirth occurs when a child is born at an unplanned time or at an unplanned place. This may happen when there is a sudden, premature delivery or when the mother cannot get to the hospital for a full-term delivery. An average pregnancy is 40 weeks. If the baby is born before the 37th week, it is considered premature. Miscarriage is the loss of the fetus before the 20th week of pregnancy.

Pregnancy and childbirth

A baby is born in a three-stage process called labour. It can be hard to tell when labour has started, but it has probably begun when one of the following happens:

- the uterus contracts at regular intervals of ten to twenty minutes, with contractions getting increasingly stronger and closer together

- amniotic fluid comes out of the vagina, which means the amniotic sac has broken—this may be called the "water breaking." There may be a trickle or a rush of fluid

- blood and mucus come from the vagina—this "bloody show" means that the mucus plug that had sealed the cervix has come out because the cervix has started to open

Stage 1: Early labour—opening of the cervix

The first stage of labour, called early labour, can take up to eighteen hours for a first child, but may be much shorter for the second or subsequent children. Usually there is enough time to get the mother to a medical facility. Early labour involves muscular contractions that may begin as an aching feeling in the lower back. As contractions get stronger, they feel like cramps in the lower abdomen. Contractions cause the cervix to open, or dilate. The cervix has to dilate until the opening is about 10 cm across before the fetus can be pushed down the birth canal, which is the second stage of labour.

Stage 2: Birth of the baby

The second stage of labour usually takes about one hour. It begins when the cervix is fully dilated and the contractions start to push the fetus out of the uterus and through the vagina. When the baby's head is close to the vaginal opening, the mother may feel a tremendous urge to push the fetus out. Usually, the fetus' head is born first, then one shoulder, then the other shoulder, and then the rest of the body is pushed out quite quickly. This second stage of labour ends when the baby is born. The baby will still be connected to the mother by the umbilical cord attached to the placenta, still in the uterus.

Stage 3: Delivery of the placenta

The third stage of labour is the delivery of the placenta after the baby is born. The uterus gets smaller and pushes the placenta out. This stage usually takes ten to twenty minutes. Labour is finished when the placenta is delivered.

7

Emergency childbirth

Your role as a first aider in emergency childbirth is to help the mother deliver the baby, to protect the mother and baby, and to save all parts of the placenta and amniotic sac until medical help takes over.

If labour is in the second stage, the baby will be born quite soon. Recognize the second stage of labour by:

- longer and stronger contractions, less than two minutes apart
- the mother's previous experience—if she says the baby is coming, believe her
- bulging of the vaginal opening and seeing the baby's head (called crowning)
- the mother is straining and pushing down, and feels like she has to have a bowel movement

If you see these signs, you will probably not have time to get the mother to medical help. Call medical help to the scene, if possible, and get ready to deliver the baby.

7

Emergency delivery

1. Locate someone to help you. Get the materials you will need to deliver the baby and the placenta.

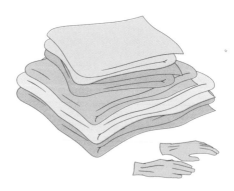

2. During the second stage of labour, when the baby will be born very soon, place the mother on her back with knees bent and head supported, unless she prefers another position. Cover her with sheets so you can easily lift them to check on the progress of labour.

3. When you can see the baby's head, the mother can push with the contractions. Tell her to wait until the contraction peaks, then take a deep breath, put her chin on her chest and push down as hard and as long as she can, while she is holding her breath. She may be able to push like this twice for each contraction. Position yourself to watch for the baby.

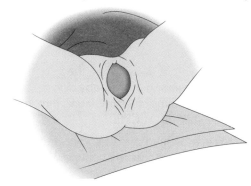

7

4. Usually the head is born first and if it comes out too quickly, the baby could be injured. As the head comes out, tell the mother to control her pushing. Support the baby as it is born, but be careful. A new-born baby has a very slippery whitish coating—handle the baby gently, firmly and carefully.

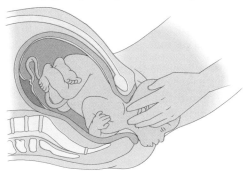

5. Clear the baby's airway—all babies have fluid in the nose and throat. Hold the baby with the head lower than the body to help drainage.

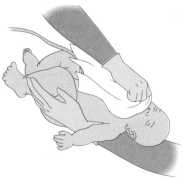

6. Most babies will cry right away. When they do, they become pink as they start breathing. If the baby doesn't start to breathe and remains pale and limp, try stimulating him. If the baby still doesn't breathe, start infant CPR.

7. Once the baby is breathing, pat them dry with a towel, being careful not to remove the slippery coating. Wrap the baby in a dry towel or blanket to keep them warm. Check the umbilical cord. If the cord is still pulsating, keep the baby at the level of the vagina. If the cord has stopped pulsating, place the baby on their side in the mother's arms with the head low to assist drainage.

8. Check the vagina for bleeding. If bleeding from the vagina is severe—act quickly. The umbilical cord must be tied because the baby's blood may be bleeding through the cord and out of the placenta. Tie the umbilical cord and keep the baby at the same level as the vagina.

9. Wait for the placenta to be delivered. This usually happens within twenty minutes of the baby's birth, but don't be surprised if it takes longer. Gently massaging the mother's lower abdomen will quicken the delivery of the placenta.

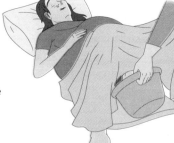

10. There may be some bleeding from the vagina after the delivery of the placenta. This is normal, and can usually be controlled by firmly massaging the uterus. The uterus can be felt as a hard, round mass in the lower abdomen. Massaging it every few minutes will help it to contract which helps control any bleeding. The baby's nursing at the mother's breast also helps to contract the uterus. Use sanitary pads to absorb any bleeding. Examine the skin between the anus and the vagina for lacerations and apply pressure with sterile dressings to any bleeding tears of the skin.

11. Give ongoing casualty care to the mother and infant. Keep them warm and comfortable and transport them to medical help as soon as possible.

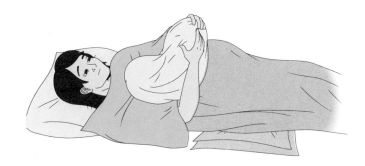

7

Vaginal bleeding and miscarriage

Miscarriage is the loss of the fetus before the 20th week of pregnancy. Most miscarriages happen because the fetus was not developing properly. The medical term for a miscarriage is spontaneous abortion.

Signs and symptoms include:

- vaginal bleeding that could be severe
- signs of shock
- cramp-like pains in the lower abdomen
- aching in the lower back
- passage of tissue

First aid for miscarriage

Your main concern in first aid for miscarriage is the shock caused by severe bleeding. The casualty may be very distressed.

1. Perform a scene survey and a primary survey. Call for medical help.

2. Give first aid for shock—place the woman on her back, or on her left side.

3. Ensure privacy. Reassure her and give her emotional support.

4. Keep any evidence of tissue and blood loss (bloody sheets, clothing, etc.). Send this with the woman to medical help for examination by the doctor.

5. Give ongoing casualty care.

7

Assault

A casualty who has been assaulted may be feeling physically and emotionally distressed. In the case of sexual assault, there may be physical injuries along with emotional ones. There is potential for the casualty to go into severe emotional shock during or shortly after the attack.

General first aid for assault

1. Perform a scene survey including obtaining consent and ensuring the scene is safe for the first aider. This is potentially an emotional situation and the casualty may be feeling vulnerable.

2. If you suspect an assault, try hard not to disturb evidence by removing, washing, or disposing of clothing.

3. Call for medical help, stay with the casualty and offer reassurance until medical help arrives.

Alcohol and Drug Considerations

7

Drugs are defined as any substance that can produce a physical or mental effect on the body. They include alcohol, prescription drugs and illegal substances. The effects of drugs are wide-ranging and can be unpredictable. Dosages and combinations of drugs (including alcohol) will affect a casualty's condition. Be prepared for behaviour which can change quickly.

First aid for a casualty on drugs or alcohol:

1. Approach the casualty in a calm, professional, sympathetic manner and try to gain their confidence.

2. Ask about the type and amount of the drug consumed, if possible.

3. If the casualty has convulsions, vomiting or low or no level of consciousness, be sure to maintain an open airway and assess breathing.

4. Give ongoing casualty care and get medical help.

5. If present, check with family members if they have been provided a medication to use in case of overdose. If available and the first aider is trained, assist with an antidote if appropriate.

Mental Health Awareness

Consider these factors and how they might affect someone:

- Critical incident or traumatic event
- Dementia in an older adult (Alzheimer disease, Lewy body disease or vascular dementia, neurocognitive disorder)
- Mood and psychiatric disorders (depression, anxiety, bipolar disorder, schizophrenia)

The World Health Organization defines health as "a state of (complete) physical, mental and social well-being and not merely the absence of disease or infirmity" (WHO). Mental health issues can be related to the health of a whole person.

There are symptoms of physical conditions that may mimic the symptoms of a mental health issue or crisis such as:

- Diabetic emergencies
- Drug reactions
- Environmental emergencies (heat and cold injuries)
- Head injuries
- Infections/fever
- Lack of oxygen
- Shock

If you are concerned for a casualty's well-being, call 911. It is more important to focus on getting the appropriate help than trying to determine a cause of the emergency.

Mental Health Continuum

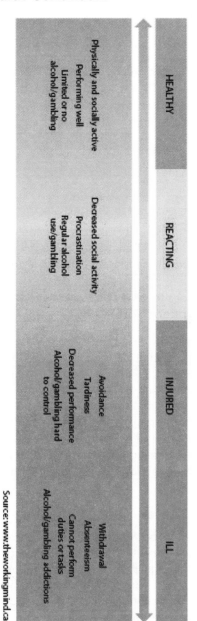

HEALTHY	REACTING	INJURED	ILL
Physically and socially active	Decreased social activity	Avoidance	Withdrawal
Performing well	Procrastination	Tardiness	Absenteeism
Limited or no alcohol/gambling	Regular alcohol use/gambling	Decreased performance	Cannot perform duties or tasks
		Alcohol/gambling hard to control	Alcohol/gambling addictions

Source: www.theworkingmind.ca

Mental Health Commission of Canada   Commission de la santé mentale du Canada

Mental Health First Aid Canada

7

The Mental Health Continuum shows the range of mental health. Those with mental health illness or mental health problems can move through this range, and with self-care, support or treatment, they can "get back to green". The focus is behaviours because loved ones or colleagues who are suffering will show certain behaviours. They can be directed to resources. **This is not a tool for diagnosing someone. That is for mental health professionals.**

CARE - Responding to a Mental Health Issue or Crisis

C – Call for help if the person is at risk of suicide

    a. If you think this is a life-threatening emergency call 911; this is a time to take action.

    b. If no risk of suicide, proceed to the next step

A – Ask & Listen. Ask the casualty how they are feeling and listen to the person's responses. The casualty may try to tell you what they need, so listening and really hearing this person is important.

R – Respond with options that may be available to them. **Important: Provide options NOT ADVICE.**

Example of what a first-aider could say, "There is a mental health crisis line that has helped other people, would you like to call them together?" Or "Maybe we could call someone that you would like to talk to (that you trust or that could help) right now?" See the Resources section for more information.

E – Encourage support in a variety of ways.

What the person may be feeling is normal and other people have felt this way too. A first aider can tell someone that they are not alone and to seek help.

Anxiety or Panic Attack

A panic or anxiety attack is both a mental health as well as a physical health issue. An anxiety attack has similar signs and symptoms to a heart attack and a first aider might not be able to differentiate between them. The anxiety attack can be serious and if left untreated, can lead to a more serious physical condition. Therefore it is always recommended to call 911.

Signs and symptoms of an anxiety attack may include some or all of the following:
- Hyperventilating (breathing too quickly)
- Chest pain or tightness
- Trembling and sweating
- Hyperventilation, tingling hands and feet
- Nausea or vomiting

First aid for a panic attack:

- Call 911 immediately.
- Sit the casualty down in a comfortable position, preferably in a quiet area if possible.
- While waiting for medical help, and if the casualty or hyperventilating, attempt to control or slowdown the casualty's breathing. Examples that can help someone focus on their breathing include:

    o Ask them to count to 4 while breathing in, and again count to 4 while breathing out.

    o Ask them to breathe in through the nose and out through the mouth.

Do not have the casualty breathe into a paper bag. This is not effective and can make the attack worse.

Crisis Help and Other Mental Health Resources

- 9-1-1 or 2-1-1; Check your local directory if not available in your region
- Kids Help Phone 1-800-668-6868 (all ages 20 and under)
- Mental Health Helpline 1-866-531-2600 or Web Chat www.mentalhealthhelpline.ca
- **www.suicideprevention.ca** – This resource has listings for Mental Health Crisis and Suicide help by province
- Local Employee Assistance Programs
- Mental Health First Aid: A 2-day program by the Mental Health Commission of Canada.
- The Working Mind: A longitudinal program by the Mental Health Commission of Canada that focuses on resiliency in the workplace.

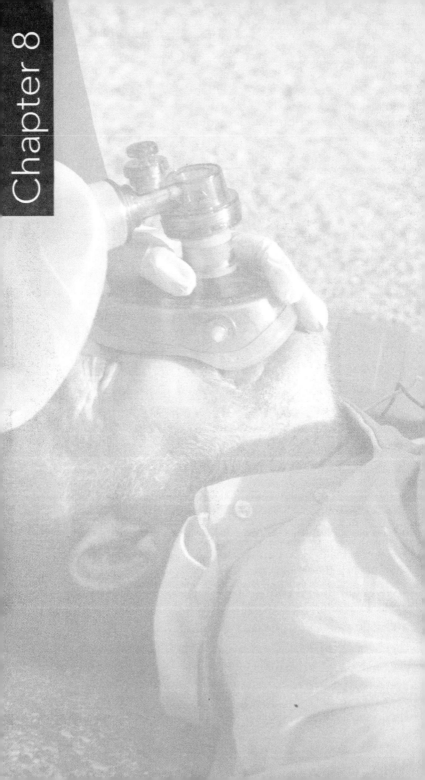

Resuscitation Skills for Health Care Providers

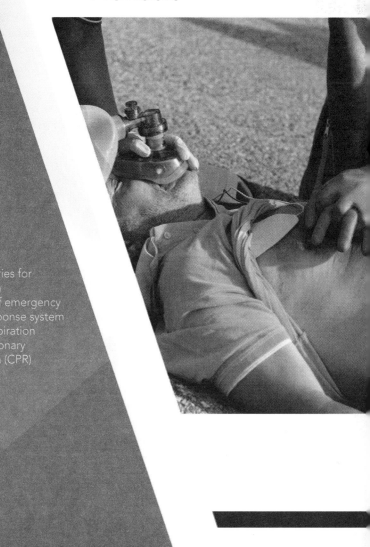

Chapter 8 Resuscitation skills for health care providers

High quality CPR includes an uninterrupted compression rate of 100-120 per minute, appropriate compression depth based on the age of the casualty and allowing for complete chest recoil after each compression.

It is important to remember that where local protocols (including legislation, medical direction and professional/workplace requirements) differ from this information, the local protocol supersedes information in this chapter.

Age categories for resuscitation

The health care provider will respond to casualties based on the following categories:

- Adult—onset of puberty and older
- Child—1 year of age to the onset of puberty (about 12 to 14 years, as defined by the presence of secondary sex characteristics)
- Infant—anyone under the age of 1 year
- Neonate/newborn—an infant who has been delivered, and in the first hours after birth and until they leave the hospital. The health care provider will not need to differentiate this group from other infants, unless they are specifically trained to provide resuscitative care for that age group.

Activation of emergency medical response system

Health care providers should be familiar with when and how to activate their own internal and/or external Emergency Medical Response system. A plan should be in place to allow for an AED to arrive on scene with the rescuer, or for an AED to be quickly retrieved and easily accessible.

Casualties of all age—two rescuers

Anytime two rescuers are present, one rescuer should stay and begin CPR while the second rescuer will activate the Emergency Medical Response System and obtain an AED, if one is not already present.

Adult casualty—lone rescuer

Anyone in cardiac arrest will need CPR, defibrillation and Advanced Life Support.

The lone rescuer should activate the Emergency Medical Response System immediately when they encounter a witnessed arrest or an unwitnessed unresponsive adult casualty.

When a casualty of any age is believed to have suffered an asphyxial arrest, the lone rescuer should call for help using a mobile phone. The phone can be put on speaker phone to save time. If a mobile device is not present, the rescuer should provide two minutes of CPR before leaving to activate EMS and obtaining the AED. The objective is to correct the cause of the arrest, the lack of oxygen, by performing two minutes of CPR first.

8

Infant and child casualty—lone rescuer

When the lone rescuer witnesses a child or infant casualty who suddenly collapses they should immediately activate their Emergency Medical Response System and obtain and use the AED right away. In the case of an unwitnessed casualty, if they cannot activate the Emergency Medical Response System from the scene, the lone rescuer should provide two minutes of CPR before leaving to call.

When activating the Emergency Medical Response System, the rescuer may consider carrying the infant/child if the casualty is small enough, if injuries permit and if the distance they must go does not impact on the start or resumption of CPR.

Artificial respiration

Artificial respiration (AR) is a way you can supply air to the lungs of a casualty who is breathing ineffectively or not breathing at all but has an adequate pulse. Pulse/breathing checks should be performed every two minutes for at least 5 seconds but no longer than 10 seconds.

The methods for ventilating a non-breathing casualty are:

- **mouth-to-mask with supplemental oxygen**

- **two person bag-valve mask**

Infants and children with a pulse rate of less than 60 beats per minute and who show signs of poor perfusion despite oxygen and ventilation should receive chest compressions in addition to ventilations.

Artificial respiration can be given in a wide range of situations. In an emergency situation, keep the following in mind:

- you can start AR right away in any position (but it is best if the casualty is on their back on a firm, flat surface)

- you can continue AR while the casualty is being moved to safety by other rescuers

- you can give AR for a long time without getting too tired

- AR techniques can be used to help a casualty with severe breathing difficulties

Giving AR in some situations may be more difficult than in others. Some examples are:

- when severe injuries to the mouth and nose prevent a good seal around the mouth

- when blood and/or other body fluids drain into the throat and block the airway, do your best to drain the mouth prior to beginning AR

- the casualty has been poisoned by a toxic gas-like hydrogen sulphide and coming in contact with the casualty may result in you being poisoned

- the casualty has a corrosive poison on the face or in the mouth, and you don't have a face mask

8

hen this happens, you have to do the best you can (based on
ur level of training) without putting yourself into danger.

pening the airway

ealth care providers will primarily open a casualty's airway using
e head-tilt chin-lift, except in cases where a spinal injury is
spected. In those cases, a jaw thrust is used. In the event that a
inal injury is suspected and the jaw thrust does not work, use a
ead-tilt chin-lift to open the airway.

sing a jaw thrust

1. With the head and neck supported, position your hands on
either side of the head.

2. Steady your thumbs on the cheek bones. Grasp the angle of
the jaw with the middle, ring and little fingers and lift to open
the airway.

3. If necessary, open the mouth using the index fingers.

4. Check for signs of breathing and pulse for at least 5 and up to
10 seconds while holding the airway open with the jaw thrust.

5. If there is a pulse, but no breathing, position the mask over the
casualty's face. Blow into the casualty's mouth and watch for
the chest to rise. Keep lifting the jaw to hold the airway open.

6. If there is no pulse, begin compressions and continue CPR until
an AED arrives on scene.

8

Bag-valve mask (BVM)

A bag-valve mask is a self-inflating bag with a one-way valve that face mask can be attached to. The BVM will also accept an oxyge reservoir bag. The bags come in three sizes: adult, child, and infa

Using a bag-valve mask

- After opening and securing the airway, select the correct mas size, based on the size of the casualty (adult, infant, or child).

- Position your thumbs over the top half of the mask with your index and middle fingers over the bottom half

- Place the apex of the mask over the bridge of the nose, then lower the mask over the mouth and chin. If the mask has a large round cuff surrounding a ventilation port, centre the po over the mouth

- Use your ring and little fingers to bring the jaw up to the mas

- Instruct a second rescuer to squeeze the bag with two hands, providing only enough air to make the chest rise

Using advanced airways with masks

8

When using a pocket or bag valve mask, using an advanced airway is recommended. This involves advanced skill training. If an advanced airway is not available or you are not trained on how to use it, this does not preclude you from using a pocket mask or BVM. Using one or the other without an airway is acceptable. The health care professional may be asked to assist with the bag valve mask when an advanced responder has inserted an advanced airway. Adjunct airways (oral or nasal) may be necessary in conjunction with bag-valve mask if the casualty i unresponsive

dult and child artificial respiration

wo-rescuer—BVM

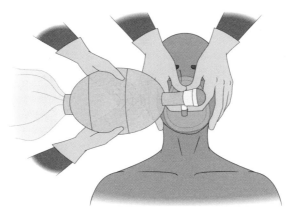

1. One rescuer positions themselves at the casualty's head, and places the mask on the face.

2. Using the thumb and first finger of EACH hand around the valve in a "C" position they press the mask against the face.

3. Using the remaining fingers of EACH hand in an "E" position they lift up on the jaw and

4. Tilt the head back to open the airway. If the casualty has a suspected head/spinal injury, use a jaw thrust.

5. The second rescuer will squeeze the bag to ventilate. Give each breath in 1 second. Make the chest visibly rise.

• adult rescue breathing: 1 breath every 5-6 sec.

• child rescue breathing: 1 breath every 3-5 sec.

6. Check the pulse approximately every 2 minutes.

8

Infant artificial respiration

Two rescuer—BVM

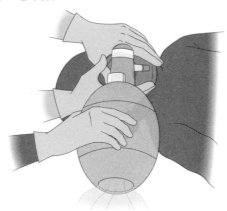

1. One rescuer positions themselves at the casualty's head and places the mask over the nose and mouth. Do not cover the eyes or chin.

2. Using the thumb and first finger of EACH hand around the valve in a "C" position they press the mask against the face.

3. Using the remaining fingers of EACH hand in an "E" position they lift up on the jaw and tilt the head back to open the airway. If the casualty has a suspected head/spinal injury, use jaw thrust.

4. The second rescuer will squeeze the bag to ventilate. Give each breath in 1 second. Make the chest visibly rise.

5. Give 1 breath every 3-5 seconds (12-20 per minute).

6. Check the pulse approximately every 2 minutes.

Assisted breathing

Assisted breathing helps a casualty with severe breathing difficulties to breathe more effectively. In a clinical setting you may have access to a CPAP (continuous positive airway pressure) machine. It is most useful when the casualty shows very little or no breathing effort. If breathing effort is good, the casualty will likely breathe better on their own. Start assisted breathing when you recognize the signs of severe breathing difficulties.

The technique for assisted breathing is the same as for artificial respiration except for the timing of the ventilations. If the casualty is breathing too slowly, give a breath each time the casualty inhales, plus an extra breath in between the casualty's own breaths. Give one breath every five seconds for a total of 12 to 15 breaths per minute.

If the casualty is breathing too fast, give one breath on every second inhalation by the casualty. This will hopefully slow down the casualty's own breathing. Give a total of 12 to 15 breaths per minute.

If the casualty is conscious, explain what you are going to do and why. Reassure the casualty often and encourage them to try to breathe at a good rate with good depth.

Artificial respiration to someone who breathes through the neck

Some people breathe through an opening at the base of the neck. This opening, called a stoma, is the result of a previous medical operation called a laryngectomy.

You may not know a person breathes through the neck when you try to give AR. If the air seems to go down the airway when you blow, but the chest doesn't rise, check the neck for a stoma. You may also hear air coming out of the stoma as you blow.

8

Giving AR to a neck breather

The first aid rescue sequence does not change. Once you recognize a person breathes through a stoma, do the following:

- expose the entire neck and remove all coverings over the stoma. If there is a tube coming out of the stoma, don't remove it

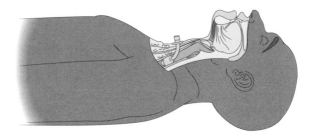

- put a pad under the shoulders to keep them slightly elevated (if you have one close by)

- keep the head in line with the body and keep the chin raised

- seal the mouth and nose with the hand closest to the head

- seal your face shield or your pocket mask over the stoma, or connect your BVM to the tracheostomy tube, and ventilate

- watch the chest rise (look, listen and feel for air movement)

- let the air escape from the stoma between breaths

- maintain a clean air passage, using a cloth to clean the opening; never use paper tissues

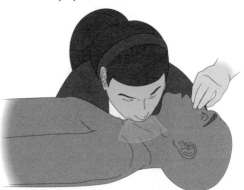

Gastric distension

If you blow into a casualty too fast or too hard, air may be bypassed into the stomach causing it to fill with air and become bloated. This is called gastric distension, and it can make it harder to ventilate the casualty and increase the chances that the casualty will vomit.

If the stomach becomes distended, try to prevent further distension by:

- repositioning the head and opening the airway again
- blowing more slowly, with less air
- making sure the airway is held fully open

It is unusual, but the stomach can become so distended that the lungs cannot expand. In this case, the air you blow won't go into the lungs, so you have to relieve the gastric distension by forcing the air in the stomach out. Only relieve gastric distension when the lungs cannot expand and AR is ineffective.

To prevent gastric distension

- give breaths at the recommended rate
- only blow enough air to make the chest rise
- make sure the airway is fully open—keep the head tilted well

8

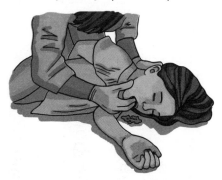

back (but not over-extended)

Cardiopulmonary resuscitation (CPR)

When assessing the casualty, the HCP will check for breathing and a pulse simultaneously before beginning compressions.

Rescuers should check the:

Adult—carotid pulse

Child—carotid or femoral pulse

Infant—brachial or femoral pulse

Brachycardia (slow pulse rate)

An infant or child with a pulse rate of less than 60 beats per minute and showing signs of poor perfusion/circulation, despite oxygen and ventilation, should also receive chest compressions. The low heart rate (<60 bpm) does not provide enough circulation to sustain adequate cellular oxygenation; by providing a compression rate of 100 to120 compressions per minute the health care provider will assist in providing adequate circulation to a casualty.

CPR (compression and ventilation) rates

8

Health care providers will provide the same compression to ventilation rates as the lay rescuer when performing one rescuer CPR for adults, children and infants; as well as two-rescuer adult, but the ratio will change when they perform two-rescuer CPR for the child and infant.

For two-rescuer CPR on a child or infant, the rescuer will provide compressions and ventilations at a ratio of 15 compressions to 2 ventilations. Depth of compressions should be at least 1/3 the depth of the infant or child's chest with a rate of 100 to 120 compressions per minute.

In the case of the infant casualty, the rescuer may encircle the infant casualty's chest and use their thumbs side-by-side or one on top of the other to provide compressions. The method used will depend on the size of the infant casualty and the rescuer's thumbs.

Adult CPR/AED

Check breathing and pulse for at least 5 and no more than 10 seconds. If there is a pulse, but no breathing, begin artificial respiration. If there is no pulse and no breathing, or only agonal breaths, begin compressions.

Agonal breathing is an abnormal pattern of breathing driven by a brainstem reflex, characterized by irregular gasping respirations at times accompanied by strange vocalizations. They can occur with cardiac arrest and lead bystanders to believe the casualty is breathing.

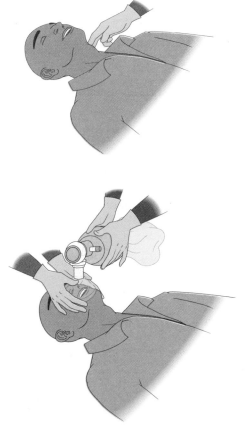

8

One rescuer 30:2

1. Give 30 chest compressions in the middle of the upper chest using two hands.

2. Push hard, push fast (100 to 120 per min) to a depth of 5-6 cm (2-2.4 inches). The pressure and release phases take the same time. Release pressure and completely remove your weight at the top of each compression to allow chest to return to the resting position after each compression. Minimize interruptions.

3. Give 2 breaths.

4. Continue 30:2 until:

   - an AED is ready for use

   - EMS/advanced providers arrive or

   - the casualty shows signs of recovery.

Two or more rescuers 30:2

1. Rescuer one—30 chest compressions at a rate of 100 to 120 per minute.

2. Rescuer two—give 2 rescue breaths, enough to make the chest visibly rise. Minimize interruptions.

3. Quickly change positions every 5 cycles (2 minutes).

4. If an advanced airway is in place—one breath every 6-8 seconds with no pause in compressions for breaths.

8

Defibrillation

1. Expose the chest. Turn on the AED. Follow the voice prompts. Select and attach the adult pads.

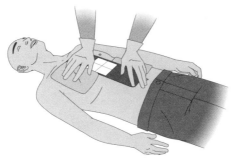

2. SHOCK advised—CLEAR and give 1 shock. Immediately resume chest compressions.

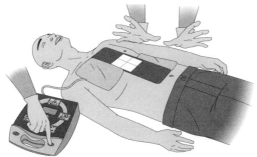

3. NO SHOCK advised—immediately resume chest compressions.

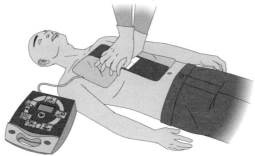

4. Continue 30 compressions—2 breaths for 5 cycles (approximately 2 minutes). Analyse heart rhythm, continue CPR/AED until advanced providers take over.

Child CPR/AED

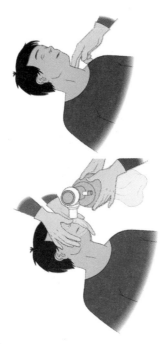

8

One rescuer 30:2

1. Give 30 chest compressions in the middle of the upper chest using one or two hands.

2. Push hard, push fast (100 to 120 per min) to a depth of about 2 inches (5 cm), or about 1/3 of the depth of the chest. The pressure and release phases take the same time. Release pressure and completely remove your weight at the top of each compression to allow chest to return to the resting position after each compression. Minimize interruptions

3. Give 2 breaths.

4. Continue 30 compressions: 2 breaths.

Two or more rescuers 15:2

1. Rescuer one—15 chest compressions at a rate of at least 100 to 120 per minute.

2. Rescuer two—give 2 rescue breaths, enough to make the chest visibly rise.

3. Quickly change positions every 10 cycles (2 minutes).

4. If an advanced airway is in place—one breath every 6-8 seconds with no pause in compressions.

Defibrillation

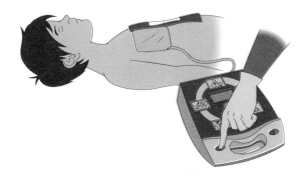

1. Expose the chest. Turn on the AED. Follow the voice prompts. Select and attach the pediatric pads. If pediatric pads are not available, use adult pads.

2. SHOCK advised: CLEAR and give 1 shock. Immediately resume chest compressions.

3. NO SHOCK advised: Immediately resume chest compressions.

4. Continue 15 compressions—2 breaths for 5 cycles (approximately 2 minutes). Analyse heart rhythm, continue CPR/AED until advanced providers take over.

8

Infant CPR/AED

In the case of the infant casualty, the rescuer may encircle the infant casualty's chest and use their thumbs side-by-side or one on top of the other to provide compressions. The method used will depend on the size of the infant casualty and the rescuer's thumbs.

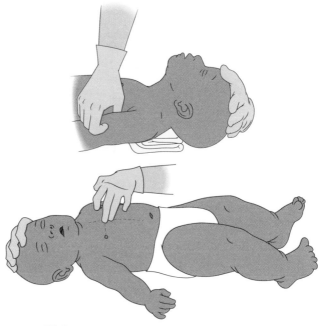

One rescuer 30:2

1. Give 30 chest compressions just below the nipple line using two fingers.

2. Push hard, push fast (100 to 120 per minute) to a depth of about 1 1/2 inches (4 cm) or 1/3 of the depth of the chest. The pressure and release phases take the same time. Release pressure and completely remove your weight at the top of each compression to allow chest to return to the resting position after each compression. Minimize interruptions.

3. Give 2 breaths.

4. Continue 30 compressions: 2 breaths.

Two or more rescuers 15:2

1. Rescuer one—15 chest compressions at a rate of at least 100 to 120 per minute.

2. Rescuer two—give 2 rescue breaths, enough to make the chest visibly rise.

3. Quickly change positions every 10 cycles (2 minutes).

4. If an advanced airway is in place—one breath every 6-8 seconds with no pause in compressions.

Defibrillation

1. Expose the chest. Turn on the AED. Follow the voice prompts. Select and attach the pediatric pads. If pediatric pads are not available, use adult pads.

2. SHOCK advised: CLEAR and give 1 shock. Immediately resume chest compressions.

3. NO SHOCK advised: Immediately resume chest compressions.

4. Continue 15 compressions—2 breaths for 5 cycles (approximately 2 minutes). Analyse heart rhythm, continue CPR/AED until advanced providers take over.

Team approach

8

Health care providers should practice working in integrated teams. When a team is available, one rescuer provides airway control and ventilations right away, a second rescuer begins compressions and a third obtains and uses the AED. This is the optimal situation as the rescuers have the ability to maximize the compression fraction of CPR prior to defibrillation. A high performance team can achieve compression fractions of 80%, i.e. perform effective chest compression for the majority of the time they are resuscitating the casualty.

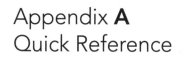

Appendix **A**
Quick Reference

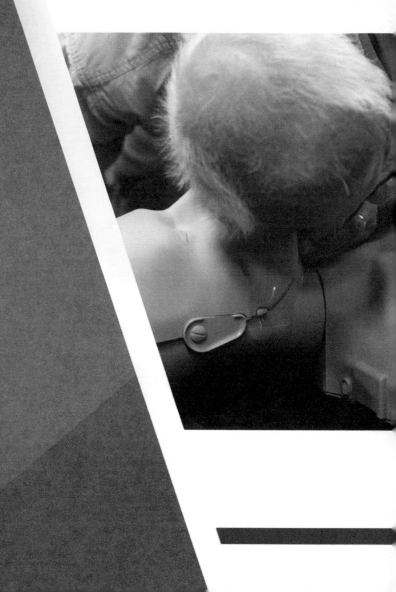

SAMPLE FIRST AID REPORT

Unit ID   CALL NUMBER

Patient :

Surname: _____ Given Names: _____ Date of Birth: _____ Sex: M F

Contact Information: _____ _____ Telephone: _____
_____

Details of the Illness/Injury

Date: _____ and Time: _____ am/pm Location: _____

Patient found: Ambulatory: ☐ Sitting: ☐   Prone: ☐ Supine: ☐ Side: Left ☐ Right ☐

Patient brought in by: Self: ☐ Staff: ☐ Co-worker: ☐ Other: ☐ Name: _____

LOC: Alert: ☐ Verbal: ☐ Pain: ☐ Unresponsive: ☐

Chief Complaint::

Symptoms
(OPQRST)

Allergies
Medications
Previous Hx
Last Oral Intake
Events Prior

Vital Signs Record	Time	Time	Time		Assessment
Blood Pressure					
Pulse					**A**brasion
Breathing					**B**urn
Skin					**C**ontusion
Pupils					**D**eformity
SpO2					**F**racture
Blood Glucose					**H**aemorrhage
Treatment Provided:					**L**aceration
Oxygen:					**P**ain
					Rigidity
					Swelling
					Tenderness

Follow Up/Referral - None ☐ Nurse ☐ Doctor ☐ Ambulance ☐ Hospital ☐ Other ☐ _____

Refusal of Care: I _____ do not wish to receive medical/first aid care from these First Responders. I have been advised that I need medical/first aid care and have decided to refuse it. I do not hold the first responders and their parent agency responsible for any negative consequences that I may suffer from this refusal.

Signature of patient: _____ Signature of witness: _____

First Aid Attendant (Print):	Time:
Signature:	Date:
First Aid Attendant (Print):	Time:
Signature:	Date:

274

Quick first aid reference

Send for an ambulance as soon as there is indication of a life-threatening emergency:

- loss of consciousness
- breathing emergency (difficult or stopped breathing)
- circulatory emergency (severe bleeding, heart attack, stroke)

Signs and symptoms   First aid

Allergic reaction

Signs and symptoms	First aid
Itchy, flushed skin	Position casualty at rest
Sneezing, runny nose	If casualty has medication, help her to take it
Swelling of the airway	Monitor the ABCs
Nausea, vomiting	Get medical help

Angina

Signs and symptoms	First aid
Denial, sense of impending doom	Position casualty at rest
Heaviness, tightness in chest	If casualty has medication, help her to take it
Indigestion, aching jaw	Monitor the ABCs
Pale skin, sweating	Get medical help

Asthma

Signs and symptoms	First aid
Shortness of breath with coughing or wheezing	Position casualty for comfort sitting or semi-sitting
Sitting upright, trying to breathe	Assist with medication
Blue colour to face (cyanosis)	Monitor the ABCs
Anxiety, tightness in chest	Get medical help

Bites and stings

Signs and symptoms	First aid
Pain at site	Position casualty at rest
Heat and swelling at site	Remove stinger if appropriate
Redness, itching	Clean affected area
Rash or bumps on skin	Monitor the ABCs

A

Bleeding (external)

Obvious wound

Apply pressure

External blood

Position casualty at rest

Cold, clammy skin

Apply dressings and bandages

Restlessness, apprehension

Check circulation before and after bandaging

Faintness, dizziness

Bleeding (internal)

No obvious wound

Shock position, if injuries permit

Blood from ears, nose, in urine/stool

If thirsty, moisten lips

Bloodshot or black eye(s)

Monitor the ABCs

Blood coughed up or in vomitus

Get medical help

Burns

Skin red to pearly white or charred

Position casualty at rest

Pain in mild cases, no pain if severe

Cool the affected area

Blisters

Apply dressings and bandages

Moist skin, dry leathery if severe

Check circulation

Choking

Mild obstruction

Stay with casualty

Able to speak

Encourage casualty to cough

Signs of distress

If obstruction not cleared, get medical help

Red face

Severe obstruction

Position yourself supporting the casualty

Not able to speak

Give 5 back blows, 5 abdominal thrusts

Weak or no coughing

Be prepared for loss of consciousness

Grey face, blue lips, ears

Concussion

Partial or complete loss of consciousness usually of short duration

If you suspect head/spinal injury, do not move casualty

Shallow breathing, nausea

Monitor the ABCs

Pale, sweating, headache

Get medical help

A

Diabetic emergency

Hypoglycemia (needs sugar)

   Sweaty, pale, cold

   Headache, trembling

   Confusion, irritable, aggressive

Hyperglycemia (needs insulin)

   Flushed, dry, warm

   Drowsy, becoming unconscious

   Thirsty, breath smells like nail polish

Position casualty at rest

Give sugar

Monitor the ABCs

If no improvement, get medical help

Position casualty at rest

If unsure, whether hyper or hypo, give sugar

Monitor the ABCs

Get medical help

Embedded object

   Obvious wound

   Object visible in wound

   (Do not remove embedded object)

   Bleeding at wound site

Position casualty at rest

Build up dressings around object

Apply dressings without pressure on object

Bandage get medical help

Emergency childbirth

   Longer and stronger contractions

   Mother tells you the baby is coming

   Straining, bearing down

   Feeling she has to have bowel movement

Position casualty at rest

Keep casualty warm

Place sanitary napkin or clean pad for bleeding

Get medical help

Fainting

   Pale, sweaty

   Dizzy and nauseous

   Unsteady, may collapse

Position casualty at rest

Loosen tight clothing, get fresh air

Stay with casualty until fully recovered

Frostbite

   White waxy skin

   Skin firm but soft underneath

   Skin becomes cold and hard

   Painful at first, then numb

Get casualty out of cold

Position casualty

If frostbite is superficial, rewarm the area

Give first aid for wounds

A

Head/spinal injury

Confused, lightheaded

Mechanism of injury to suggest

Pale, cold, clammy

Tell casualty not to move

Monitor the ABCs

Get medical help

Heart attack (see Angina)

Denial, sense of impending doom

Heaviness, tightness in chest

Indigestion, aching jaw

Pale skin, sweating

Unconsciousness

Stopped breathing

If conscious, position casualty at rest

If casualty has medication, help her to take it

Monitor the ABCs

Get medical help

If unresponsive and not breathing,

get medical help, and send for AED

Begin CPR

Hypothermia

Shivering gets worse, then stops

Breathing slows, and may stop

Confused, sleepy, irrational
may lose consciousness

Get casualty out of cold

Position casualty at rest

Only rewarm a casualty with mild hypothermia

Get medical help

Heat exhaustion

Excessive sweating, dilated pupils

Dizziness, blurred vision, headache, cramps

Cold, clammy skin, shallow breathing

Possible loss of consciousness

Get casualty out of heat

Give as much to drink as she will take

Remove excessive clothing

Monitor the ABCs

Heatstroke

Body temperature hot to touch

Skin flushed, hot and may be wet or dry

Restless, headache, dizziness

Vomiting, convulsions, unconsciousness

Cool the casualty

Remove excess clothing

Immersion in cold water

Get medical help

Poisoning

Swallowed

    nausea, vomiting,

    discolouration at lips, burns

Absorbed

    Red skin, blisters, swelling, burns

Injected Monitor consciousness and breathing

    Irritation at point of entry

Inhaled

    Trouble breathing, chest pain

Position casualty

Conscious casualty - call Poison Control

Unconscious casualty - get medical help

If powder, brush off

Flush area with large amounts of water

Monitor the ABCs

Ensure safety of yourself and others

Get medical help.

Seizure

    Sudden cry

    Stiffening of body

    Loss of consciousness, causing
    casualty to fall

    Breathing irregular or stopped

    Loss of bladder or bowel control

Do not interfere during seizure

Protect casualty from injury

When the seizure has ended,
place the unconscious casualty
into the recovery position

Monitor the ABCs

Get medical help

Stroke

    F.A.S.T.

    Complains of sudden weakness

    Symptoms related to affected area

    Dizziness, headache

Position conscious casualty at rest

Give nothing by mouth

Monitor the ABCs

Get medical help

Unconsciousness

    Eyes do not open

    Does not respond to instructions

    Does not respond to touch

    Indicates worsening of existing
    condition

Get medical help

Give first aid for injuries or illness

Position casualty in recovery position

Monitor the ABCs

A

Cardiopulmonary resuscitation

Assess responsiveness

If unresponsive, send someone to call for medical help and get an AED. Check breathing for at least 5 and not more than 10 seconds. If not breathing:

Begin compressions

Adult

Use two hands

Child

Use one or two hands

Infant

Use two fingers

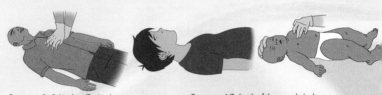

Compress 2 - 2.4 inches (5 - 6cm)

Compress 1/3 depth of the casualty's chest

Push hard, push fast

- Compress at a rate of 100-120 per minute
- Give 30 compressions
- Open airway and give two breaths
- Continue CPR at ratio of 30 compressions to two breaths until:

  - medical help arrives
  - someone else takes over, or
  - you are to exhausted to continue

Additional rescue carries

The most common carries are presented in Chapter 2 in the section on Lifting and Carrying. In some cases, these carries may not be appropriate. Additional carries are presented here. Always be aware of the risk to both the first aider and the casualty, and the increased danger if a casualty suddenly loses consciousness.

Pick-a-back

This carry is used for a conscious casualty with lower limb injuries, provided he can use his arms. The casualty must be able to help get into position on your back or be already seated at chair or table height.

1. Crouch with your back between the casualty's knees.

2. Have the casualty hold on around your neck.

3. Support the casualty's legs and lift. Use your leg muscles to stand up, keeping your back straight.

If the casualty is to be carried pick-a-back for a long distance, make a carrying seat.

Make a large adjustable loop from a strap or belts. Put your arm through the loop, arranging it behind your neck and down the

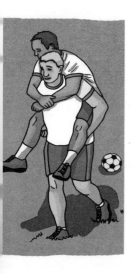

front of your shoulders. Leave the bottom half of the loop free at the back about the level of your buttocks

A

Pass the casualty's legs through the bottom of the loop; one on each side. Position the loop under the casualty's buttocks, adjusting it for a good carrying position and proper weight distribution.

Cradle carry

Use the cradle carry to lift children and lightweight adults.

1. Kneel on one knee at the casualty's side.

2. Place the casualty's arm around your neck as you support the back and shoulders.

3. Pass your other arm under the knees to grasp the thighs.

4. Ensure a solid footing and place the feet apart for good balance.

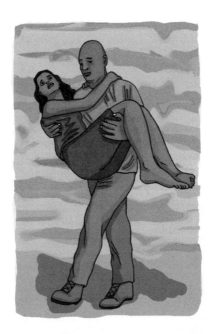

5. Lift using your legs, keep your back straight, and your abdominal muscles tense.

Fire fighter's carry

The fire fighter's carry is used for casualties who are helpless and are not too heavy for the rescuer.

1. With the casualty lying face up in front of you, stand with your toes against the casualty's toes. Grasp her wrists and pull her upward and forward.

2. Maintain a grip on one wrist as you turn and bend to catch the casualty's upper body across your shoulder. The lifting manoeuvre is a continuous, smooth motion to bring the casualty through a sitting position to an upright position, finishing with the casualty draped over your shoulder.

3. Adjust the weight across your shoulders, with the casualty's legs straddling your shoulder.

4. Pass your arm between the casualty's legs and grasp her wrist. This will stabilize the casualty on your shoulders and leave your other hand free.

Two-hand seat

A casualty, who is unable to support his upper body, can be carried by two rescuers, using the two-hand seat.

1. The rescuers crouch on either side of the casualty.

2. Each rescuer reaches across the casualty's back to grasp his clothing at the waist on the opposite side.

3. Each rescuer passes his other hand under the thighs, keeping his fingers bent and holding padding to protect against the fingernails. Hook the bent fingers together to form a rigid seat. Alternatively, the rescuers can hold each other's wrists.

A

4. The rescuers lift with their legs, keeping their backs straight. Once in the standing position, the rescuers adjust their hands and arms for comfort. When the casualty is securely positioned, the bearers step off together, each using the inside foot.

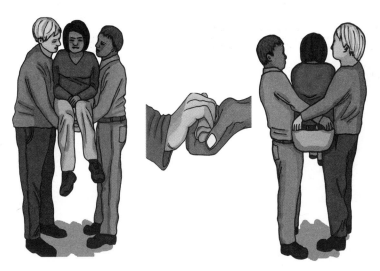

Four-hand seat

A conscious casualty who can use his hands and arms can be carried on a four-hand seat by two rescuers.

1. Each rescuer grasps his own left wrist with his right hand, then grasps the right wrist of the other rescuer with his left hand to form a square.

2. Tell the casualty to put his arms around the rescuers' shoulders and hoist himself up to permit the bearers to pass their hands under the buttocks to position them under the thighs at a point of balance.

3. Instruct the casualty to hold onto the rescuers' shoulders to keep his balance and support his upper body.

A

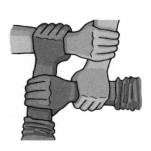

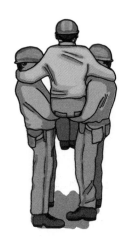

Using a blanket with a stretcher

A casualty can be wrapped on a stretcher so that a blanket provides maximum warmth with minimum weight on the casualty. It will also allow easy access to the casualty's wounds if that is necessary during transportation.

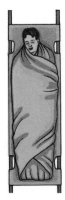

1. Place a blanket on the stretcher under the casualty with diagonally opposite corners at the head and feet.

2. Place padding at appropriate places on the blanket to fill the natural hollows at the casualty's neck and back. Centre the casualty on the blanket.

3. Cover the feet with the bottom corner and bring the corner at the head around the neck to the chest. Wrap the legs and lower body with one side. Tuck in the last corner on the opposite side.

A

Appendix **B**
The Body and
How it Works

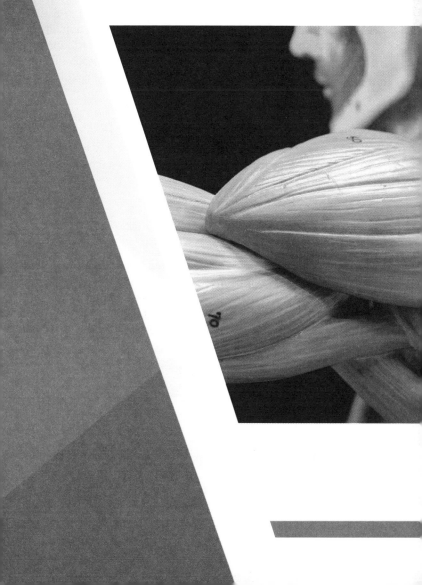

Introduction to anatomy and physiology

As a first aider, you don't need a full knowledge of anatomy and physiology. However, you should know the basic structure of the human body and how it functions normally. This chapter describes the terms used in anatomy so that you can be more precise when giving information about a person's condition. It gives a short description of the major organs and functions of the skin, musculoskeletal system, nervous system including the eye, digestive and urinary, circulatory and respiratory systems.

Anatomical terms

These are the words used to describe where things are on the body and how they relate to each other.

proximal—closer to the attachment of arm/leg: e.g., the elbow is proximal to the wrist

anterior—toward the front of the body

posterior—toward the back of the body

superior—part toward the head of the body

extension—straightening a joint

flexion—bending a joint

inferior —the part toward the feet of the body

distal—further away from the attachment of arm/leg: e.g., the fingers are distal to the wrist

lateral—away from the midline of body: e.g., the small toe is lateral to the big toe

medial—nearer to midline: e.g., the big toe is medial to the small toe

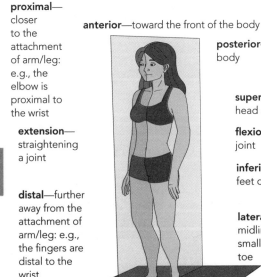

B

The skin

The skin is an important organ of the body. Its primary functions are to protect the body from environmental hazards and infection, eliminate waste in the form of sweat, help maintain normal body temperature and tell the brain of environmental temperature changes.

Environmental control

A rich supply of nerves in the skin keeps the brain aware of environmental changes. These nerves are sensitive to heat, cold, pain and touch, and they transmit these sensations to the brain. The skin helps the body adjust to its environment and protects it from extreme temperatures. In cold temperatures, blood vessels constrict to reduce blood flow near the surface of the skin. This helps prevent loss of heat from the body core. The fatty layers under the skin insulate the body to keep in body heat. In hot temperatures, the blood vessels near the skin surface dilate (get larger), allowing more blood flow near the skin. This cools the body by moving heat from the core to the surface, where it either radiates from the body, or is used to evaporate perspiration, having a cooling effect.

Functions of the skin

- to protect the body from bacterial invasion
- to help control body temperature
- to retain body fluids
- to help eliminate waste products through perspiration
- to insulate the body

B

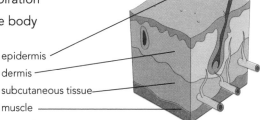

epidermis
dermis
subcutaneous tissue
muscle

Musculoskeletal system

The musculoskeletal system is the framework of the body within which organs and body systems function. This framework includes bones, muscles, tendons and ligaments. Bones act as levers for muscle action; muscles shorten to produce movement; tendons attach muscles to bones; ligaments attach bones to bones at the joints. The musculoskeletal system protects organs, supports the body, and provides for its movement.

Muscles

Muscles are made of a special kind of tissue that contracts (shortens) when stimulated by nerve impulses. Generally, body movement is caused by several muscles working in combination—as some are contracting, others are relaxing. The nerves in the muscles carry impulses to and from the brain. Muscles are classified as either voluntary or involuntary. Voluntary muscles are consciously controlled by the person, meaning they can be contracted or relaxed as the individual wishes. The muscles that move the skeleton are voluntary.

Involuntary muscles contract and relax rhythmically without any conscious effort on the part of the person. The heart, which has its own regulating system, is a good example of an involuntary muscle.

The diaphragm, a large dome-shaped muscle that separates the chest and abdominal cavities and is used in breathing, has characteristics of both voluntary and involuntary muscles. The contraction of the muscle, and thus the rate of breathing, can be changed at will for short periods of time.

B

keleton

e skeleton, made up of bones, forms the supporting
ucture that gives the body its shape. It also protects
any of the organs—for example, the brain is protected
 the skull, the heart and lungs by the ribs, and the
inal cord by the vertebrae.

e joints

e bones allow body
ovement by serving as
id levers for tendons and
uscles. The joints are
rmed where two
more bones come
gether. Immovable joints
ow no movement, as
the bones of the adult
ull. Slightly movable

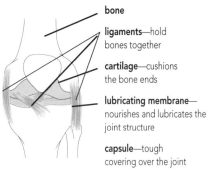

bone

ligaments—hold
bones together

cartilage—cushions
the bone ends

lubricating membrane—
nourishes and lubricates the
joint structure

capsule—tough
covering over the joint

nts allow only limited movement and are found
tween the vertebrae and between the pelvis and the
ine. Freely moving joints are covered with smooth
rtilage to minimize friction, and
 held together by bands of strong tissue called
aments.

ine

e spine is divided into five parts as shown in the
agram. There are 33 bones in the spine, called
rtebrae. The vertebrae stack on top of each other
th **discs** between them. The discs are made of a
ugh flexible material and serve as shock absorbers in
 spine. All the discs and vertebrae have an opening
 the centre such that, when they stack together,
ere is a long channel that runs from the top to the
ttom of the spine. The spinal cord, which carries all
rve impulses to and from the brain, runs through this
annel. The spine protects the spinal cord, but if the
ine is fractured, broken bones, displaced tissue and
elling can damage the spinal cord, possibly causing
elong disability.

B

Thorax

The thorax is made up of the ribs, the 12 thoracic vertebrae and the sternum (breastbone). The thorax protects the organs in the chest, mainly the heart and lungs. It also provides some protection for the upper abdominal organs, including the liver at the front and the kidney at the back. Injuries to the bones the thorax threaten the organs the protect, and can therefore be life-threatening.

Parts of the spine

cervical
7 vertebrae

thoracic
12 vertebrae

lumbar
5 vertebrae

sacral
5 fused
vertebrae

coccygeal
4 fused
vertebrae form
the tailbone

ribs —12 pairs are attached to the vertebrae in back and either to the sternum, or to each other, in front. The lowest ribs attach to the vertebrae only, and are called "floating ribs"

sternum—a dagger-shaped bone with the point downward

xiphoid process (tip of sternum)—a strong piece of cartilage. Pressure on this cartilage can damage underlying organs

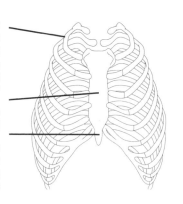

Skull

All the bones of the head make up the skull. The skull gives the head its shape and also protects the brain. When the skull fractured, the brain m also be injured.

cranium—the plate-like bones fuse together during childhood to form a rigid case for the brain

facial bones join with bones of the cranium to form the eye and nose cavities which protect the eyes and nose

upper jaw (maxilla)

lower jaw (mandible)

B

Main bones of the skeleton

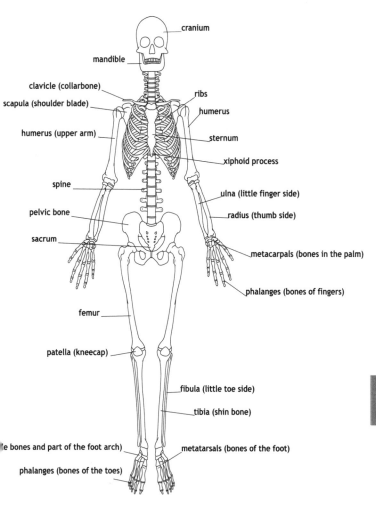

cranium

mandible

clavicle (collarbone)

scapula (shoulder blade)

ribs

humerus

humerus (upper arm)

sternum

xiphoid process

spine

ulna (little finger side)

pelvic bone

radius (thumb side)

sacrum

metacarpals (bones in the palm)

phalanges (bones of fingers)

femur

patella (kneecap)

fibula (little toe side)

tibia (shin bone)

e bones and part of the foot arch)

metatarsals (bones of the foot)

phalanges (bones of the toes)

B

Nervous system

The nervous system is composed of the brain, spinal cord and nerves. The brain and spinal cord together are called the **central nervous system**. The nerves th spread out to all parts of the body are called **peripher nerves**. The nervous system is sub divided into the **voluntary nervous system** and the **autonomic nervou system**. The voluntary nervous system controls functic at the will of the individual. The autonomic nervous system controls functions without the conscious effort of the individual—e.g. heartbeat, breathing, blood pressure, digestion and glandular secretions such as hormones.

The peripheral nerves that extend from the spinal cord to all parts of the body are of two kinds—motor nerves and sensory nerves. Motor nerves control movement. Sensory nerves transmit sensations of tou taste, heat, cold and pain to the brain.

Brain

The brain, the controlling organ of the body, occupies almost all the space in the cranium. It is the centre of consciousness, memory and thought. It receives information and transmits impulses to all parts of the body for voluntary and involuntary activities.

Eyes

The eye is the organ of sight. Any injury to the eye is potentially serious and may result in impaired vision o blindness. The quick response of the first aider and th correct first aid may help prevent permanent damage the eye.

B

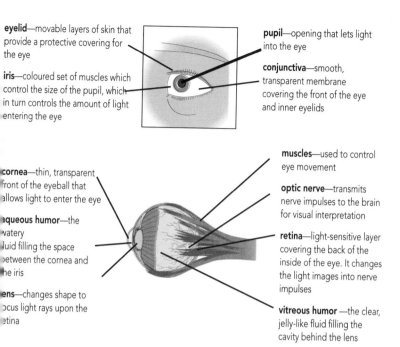

eyelid—movable layers of skin that provide a protective covering for the eye

iris—coloured set of muscles which control the size of the pupil, which in turn controls the amount of light entering the eye

pupil—opening that lets light into the eye

conjunctiva—smooth, transparent membrane covering the front of the eye and inner eyelids

cornea—thin, transparent front of the eyeball that allows light to enter the eye

aqueous humor—the watery fluid filling the space between the cornea and the iris

lens—changes shape to focus light rays upon the retina

muscles—used to control eye movement

optic nerve—transmits nerve impulses to the brain for visual interpretation

retina—light-sensitive layer covering the back of the inside of the eye. It changes the light images into nerve impulses

vitreous humor—the clear, jelly-like fluid filling the cavity behind the lens

Digestive and urinary systems

The digestive and urinary systems convert food and drink into nutrients for the cells and collect and dispose of solid and fluid waste. The organs of these systems are classified as hollow or solid. The hollow, tubular organs carry digestive and urinary materials. The solid organs are tissue masses with a rich blood supply.

Injury to hollow organs may allow the contents to spill out into the abdominal or pelvic cavities, causing infection. Injury to the solid organs can result in severe internal bleeding.

B

Digestive system

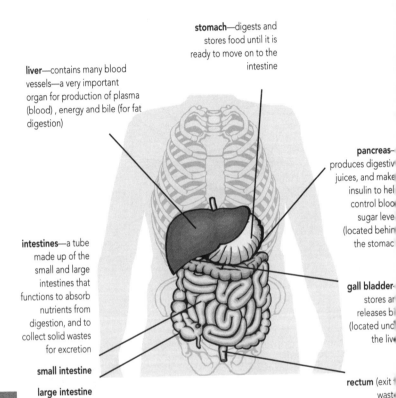

stomach—digests and stores food until it is ready to move on to the intestine

liver—contains many blood vessels—a very important organ for production of plasma (blood) , energy and bile (for fat digestion)

pancreas—produces digestiv juices, and make insulin to hel control bloo sugar leve (located behin the stomac

intestines—a tube made up of the small and large intestines that functions to absorb nutrients from digestion, and to collect solid wastes for excretion

gall bladder—stores ar releases b (located und the liv

small intestine

large intestine

rectum (exit waste

B

Urinary system

The urinary system removes and collects waste products from the blood and eliminates them from the body in the form of urine. It is made up of the kidneys, ureters, bladder and urethra.

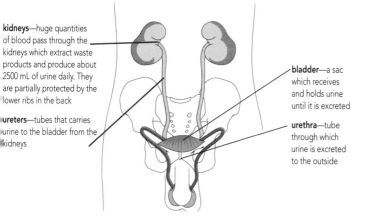

kidneys—huge quantities of blood pass through the kidneys which extract waste products and produce about 2500 mL of urine daily. They are partially protected by the lower ribs in the back

ureters—tubes that carries urine to the bladder from the kidneys

bladder—a sac which receives and holds urine until it is excreted

urethra—tube through which urine is excreted to the outside

Circulatory system

The circulatory system is a complex closed circuit consisting of the heart and blood vessels that circulates blood throughout the body. Blood circulation is essential for distributing oxygen and nutrients to cells, and for collecting waste products from cells for excretion from the body.

Heart

The heart is a hollow, muscular organ about the size of a fist. It is located in the chest cavity behind the sternum. The heart functions as a two-sided pump, continuously pumping blood to the lungs and throughout the body. It pumps by first relaxing and filling up with blood, then

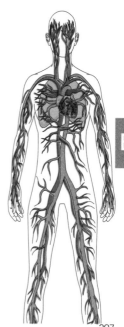

B

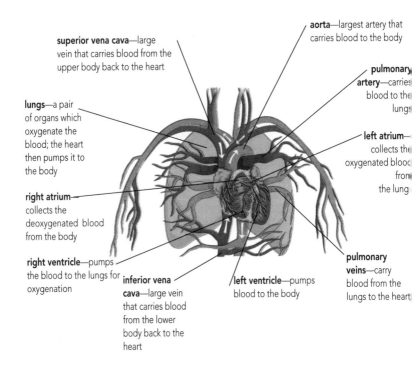

superior vena cava—large vein that carries blood from the upper body back to the heart

aorta—largest artery that carries blood to the body

pulmonary artery—carries blood to the lungs

lungs—a pair of organs which oxygenate the blood; the heart then pumps it to the body

left atrium—collects the oxygenated blood from the lung

right atrium—collects the deoxygenated blood from the body

right ventricle—pumps the blood to the lungs for oxygenation

inferior vena cava—large vein that carries blood from the lower body back to the heart

left ventricle—pumps blood to the body

pulmonary veins—carry blood from the lungs to the heart

contract-ing to squeeze or pump the blood out into the blood vessels. To make the heart beat effectively, it has a complex system of nerves. These nerves carry electrical impulses that control the beating of the heart.

Blood vessels

The blood travels through blood vessels. There are three main types of blood vessels: arteries, capillaries and veins. The **arteries** are the strongest blood vessels. They carry blood, under pressure, from the heart to all parts of the body. The arteries expand according to the volume of blood being forced through them by the pumping action of the heart, and return to normal size as the heart refills for the next contraction. This pressure wave can be felt as a pulse.

The largest artery, the aorta, emerges from the top of the heart. The coronary arteries branch off from the top of the aorta to supply the heart with blood. The smallest arteries are called arterioles and eventually form **capillaries**.

Capillaries are the tiny blood vessels that reach every living cell to deliver oxygen, food, etc. and collect waste products. They have very thin walls to allow for the exchange of fluids and gases. Capillaries eventually join to form tiny venules, which in turn form veins. The **veins** take the blood back to the heart. Veins have thinner walls than arteries and most have cuplike valves that allow blood to flow only toward the heart.

Blood

Blood is the fluid that circulates through the heart and blood vessels. It transports oxygen and nutrients to the cells and carries away carbon dioxide and other waste products. Blood is composed of plasma, red cells, white cells and platelets—see sidebar.

Blood circulation

The blood circulation system is a closed loop beginning and ending at the heart. It consists of:

pulmonary circulation—starting at the right side of the heart, blood is pumped to the lungs, where it drops off carbon dioxide and picks up oxygen, and then moves it back to the left side of the heart

systemic circulation—starting at the left side of the heart, blood is pumped to the body, where it delivers oxygen and picks up carbon dioxide, and then moves it back to the right side of the heart

B

Blood components

- plasma—pale yellow liquid that carries cells, platelets, nutrients and hormones
- red blood cells—carry oxygen
- white blood cells—protect the body against microbes
- platelets—help form blood clots to stop bleeding

Blood pressure

Blood pressure is the pressure of the blood pushing against the inside walls of the blood vessels. With each heartbeat, there is a wave of pressure that travels throughout the circulatory system. The pressure wave is strong enough to be felt as a pulse at various points in the body, including
the wrist (radial pulse), the neck (carotid pulse), and the upper arm (brachial pulse). Three factors control blood pressure:

- blood volume (how much blood is in the body)
- the capacity and elasticity of the blood vessels
- the strength of the heartbeat

If blood pressure is too low, the body's tissues don't get enough oxygen. This results in shock. Severe bleeding reduces the blood volume, which affects blood pressure. The body tries to compensate for blood loss by constricting the blood vessels and reducing the capacity of the circulatory system. With continued blood loss, however, the body
cannot compensate and blood pressure drops.

B

Respiratory system

The respiratory system causes air to be drawn in and out of the lungs. The fresh air we breathe contains about 21% oxygen. In the lungs, blood picks up some of the oxygen and releases carbon dioxide. The air we breathe out has less oxygen (about 16%) and more carbon dioxide.

The respiratory system has three main parts: the airway, the lungs and the diaphragm. The airway is the passage which air follows to get from the nose and mouth to the lungs. In the lungs, blood drops off carbon dioxide and picks up oxygen. This process is called **gas exchange**. The diaphragm, a smooth, flat muscle just below the lungs, is used in breathing.

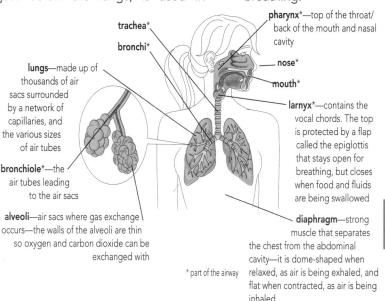

trachea*

bronchi*

lungs—made up of thousands of air sacs surrounded by a network of capillaries, and the various sizes of air tubes

bronchiole*—the air tubes leading to the air sacs

alveoli—air sacs where gas exchange occurs—the walls of the alveoli are thin so oxygen and carbon dioxide can be exchanged with

pharynx*—top of the throat/ back of the mouth and nasal cavity

nose*

mouth*

larnyx*—contains the vocal chords. The top is protected by a flap called the epiglottis that stays open for breathing, but closes when food and fluids are being swallowed

diaphragm—strong muscle that separates the chest from the abdominal cavity—it is dome-shaped when relaxed, as air is being exhaled, and flat when contracted, as air is being inhaled

* part of the airway

B

Respiratory control

Breathing is controlled by the respiratory centre in the brain, located near the base of the neck. It monitors the amount of oxygen and carbon dioxide in the blood. As the levels of oxygen and carbon dioxide change, the respiratory centre responds by changing the rate and depth of breathing.

How much oxygen is used, and how much carbon dioxide is given off, is related to the level of physical activity of the person. As physical activity goes up, more oxygen is used and more carbon dioxide is given off, so the respiratory centre increases the rate and depth of breathing to compensate (the heart rate also goes up). Breathing slows down when less oxygen is needed and less carbon dioxide is being produced.

Mechanism of breathing

The lungs have no way of drawing air into themselves. Instead, the diaphragm and the muscles between the ribs work together to expand the chest, which in turn expands the lungs. This causes air to be pulled into the lungs. As the breathing muscles relax, the chest returns to its smaller size and air is forced out of the lungs.

The lungs are covered with a smooth, slippery tissue called the pleural membrane. It is a continuous, double-layered tissue, one layer attached to the lungs and the other to the inside of the chest wall. The **pleura** acts as a lubricating layer to allow easy movement between the chest wall and the lungs, and to ensure that the lungs expand with the action of the chest wall.

B

Glossary

A

Abandonment: a first aider leaves the casualty without consent and without the care of a responsible person.

Abdominal thrust: the Heimlich manoeuvre; the manual thrusts to create pressure to expel an airway obstruction.

ABCs: Acronym meaning A= airway; B = breathing; C= circulation.

Abortion: the premature expulsion from the uterus of the products of conception.

Abrasion: a scraped or scratched skin wound.

Acute: a condition that comes on quickly, has severe symptoms and lasts a relatively short time.

Adam's apple: the bump on the front surface of the neck formed by part of the larynx (voice-box).

AED: automated external defibrillator- a device used to deliver a shock to help restart a stopped heart.

AIDS.: **acquired immunodeficiency syndrome**; a fatal disease spread through the HIV (human immunodeficiency virus).

Airway: the route for air in and out of the lungs.

Allergens: substances which trigger an allergic reaction in the body.

Allergic reaction: a hypersensitive response of the body's immune system to a particular allergen

Alveoli: air sacs of the lungs.

Amniotic sac: a sac holding fluid surrounding a fetus in the uterus,

Amputation: complete removal of an appendage (leg, arm, finger, etc.).

Anaphylaxis: serious, potentially life-threatening allergic reaction.

Anatomy: the structure of the body.

Angina (pectoris): a spasmodic pain in the chest due to a lack of blood supply to the heart.

Aorta: the largest artery in the body; originates at the left ventricle.

Aqueous humor: the watery fluid produced in the eye and located between the lens and the cornea.

Arteries: blood vessels that carry blood away from the heart.

Arteriosclerosis: a name for several conditions that cause the walls of the arteries to become thick, hard and inelastic.

ASA: acetylsalicylic acid—a medication available without prescription used to relieve pain, reduce swelling, reduce fever, etc.

Asthma: attacks of difficult breathing with wheezing/coughing, often due to allergens.

Atherosclerosis: a form of arteriosclerosis caused by fat deposits in the arterial walls.

Aura: a sensation of an impending seizure; may be a smell, taste, etc.

Autonomic nervous system: part of the nervous system that regulates involuntary functions (not controlled by conscious thought), such as pulse, breathing, digestion, hormone secretion, etc.

Avulsion: an injury where a piece of tissue is partially or completely torn away.

B

Back blows: sharp blows to the back, done to relieve an airway obstruction.

Bacteria: germs which can cause disease.

Bandage: material which holds a dressing in place.

Basic life support (BLS): maintaining the ABCs without equipment (excluding barrier devices)

Blood clot: a semi-solid mass of blood products used by the body to stop bleeding.

Blood pressure: the pressure of blood against the walls of arterial blood vessels.

Blood volume: the total amount of blood in the heart and the blood vessels.

Bloody show: the mucous and bloody discharge signalling the beginning of labour.

Brachial pulse: pulse felt on the inner upper arm, normally taken on infants.

Breech birth: the delivery of a baby's buttocks or a foot first, instead of the head.

Bronchi: the main branches of the trachea carrying air into the lungs. Smaller branches called bronchioles.

Bronchospasm: severe tightening of the bronchi/bronchioles.

Bruise: broken blood vessels under the skin.

C

Capillaries: very small blood vessels that link the arteries and the veins; allow gases and nutrients to move into and out of the tissues.

Carbon dioxide (CO$_2$): a waste gas produced by the cells; an important stimulant for control of breathing.

Carbon monoxide (CO): a dangerous, colourless, odourless gas which displaces the carrying of oxygen by the red blood cells.

Cardiovascular disease: refers to disorders of the heart and blood vessels; e.g. high blood pressure and arteriosclerosis.

Cardiac arrest: the sudden stopping of cardiac function with no pulse, and unresponsiveness.

Carotid artery: the main artery of the neck; used to assess the carotid pulse.

Carpals: small bones of the wrist.

Cartilage: a tough, elastic tissue covering the surfaces where bones meet, also forms part of the nose, and ears.

Central nervous system: part of the nervous system consisting of the brain and the spinal cord.

Cerebrovascular accident (CVA): stroke; sudden stopping of circulation to a part of the brain.

Cervical collar: a device used to immobilize and support the neck.

Cervix: the lowest portion, or neck, of the uterus.

Chest thrusts: a series of manual thrusts to the chest to relieve an airway obstruction.

Cholesterol: a fatty substance found in animal tissue or products; also produced by the body; thought to contribute to arteriosclerosis.

Chronic: a condition with a long and/or frequent occurrence.

Chronic obstructive pulmonary disease (COPD): a term describing a group of lung diseases that cause obstructive problems in the airways: usually consists of chronic bronchitis, emphysema.

Circulatory system: the heart and blood vessels.

Clavicles: the collarbones.

Clonic phase: describes a convulsion where tightness and relaxation follow one another.

Closed wound: wound where the skin is intact.

Compression: is a condition of excess pressure on some part of the brain, usually caused by a buildup of fluids inside the skull.

Concussion: a temporary disturbance of brain function usually caused by a blow to the head or neck.

Congestive heart failure: failure of the heart to pump effectively, causing a back-up of fluid in the lungs and body tissues.

Conjunctiva: the transparent membrane covering the front of the eyeball (cornea) and the inner eyelids.

Contamination: contact with dirt, microbes , etc.

Contract: to shorten; usually refers to a muscle which exerts a pull when it shortens.

Convection: the loss of heat caused by the movement of air over the body.

COPD: Chronic obstructive pulmonary disease (see above).

Cornea: the transparent front part of the eyeball.

Coronary artery: vessel which feeds the heart muscle.

Cranium: the part of the skull covering the brain.

Crepitus: the grating noise made when fractured bone ends rub together.

Croup: a group of viral infections that cause swelling of
the inner throat.

Cyanosis: a bluish or gray colour of the skin due to insufficient oxygen in the blood.

D

Decapitation: the traumatic removal of the head.

Defibrillation: applying an electrical shock to a fibrillating heart.

Deoxygenated blood: blood containing a low level of oxygen.

Dermis: the inner layer of the skin containing hair germinating cells, sweat glands, nerves and blood vessels.

Diabetes: a disease caused by insufficient insulin in the blood; causes excessive blood sugar.

Diaphragm: a large dome-shaped muscle separating the chest and abdominal cavities.

Diarrhea: excessive watery bowel movements.

Direct pressure: force applied directly on a wound to help stop bleeding.

Dislocation: when the bone surfaces at a joint are no longer in proper contact.

Distal: refers to a part that is farther away from the attachment of a leg/arm/finger/toe.

Dressing: a covering over a wound, used to stop bleeding and prevent contamination of the wound.

E

Embedded object: an object stuck onto the surface (usually on the eye) or impaled into tissues.

Embolus: any foreign matter such as a blood clot, fat clump or air bubble carried in the blood stream.

Emetic: a substance used to cause vomiting.

EMS.: emergency medical services system—a community's group of services which respond to emergencies including police, fire fighters, paramedics.

Emphysema: a chronic lung disease characterized by overstretched alveolar walls. See COPD.

Epidermis: The outermost layer of the skin.

Epiglottis: a lid-like piece of tissue which protects the entrance to the larynx (voice-box).

Epiglottitis: an infection usually in children resulting in a swelling of the epiglottis —may cause an airway obstruction.

Epilepsy: a chronic brain disorder characterized by recurrent convulsions.

ESM.: emergency scene management—the sequence of actions a first aider should follow to give safe and appropriate first aid.

Exhalation: expiration; breathing out.

Extrication: freeing from being trapped (usually a car collision).

F

Femur: the thigh bone.

Fibrillation: uncoordinated contractions of the heart muscle, so that the blood out-flow is almost nil.

Fibula: the bone of the lower leg on the little toe side.

Flail chest: a condition in which several ribs are broken in at least two places, allowing a free-floating segment.

Flexion: bending a joint.

First aid: the help given to an injured or suddenly ill person using readily available materials.

First aider: someone who takes charge of an emergency scene and gives first aid.

Fracture: a broken or cracked bone.

Frostbite: tissue damage due to exposure to cold.

G

Gallbladder: a sac under the liver that concentrates and stores bile; used for fat digestion.

Gastric distention: a swelling of the stomach usually with air, due to ventilating with excessive volume or force during artifical respiration .

G

Gauze: an open mesh material used for dressings.

Guarding: a tightening of the abdominal muscles when the casualty has abdominal pain and is touched there.

H

Head-tilt chin-lift manoeuvre: opening the casualty's airway by tilting the head backward and lifting the chin forward.

Heart attack: the damaging or death of an area of the heart muscle caused by loss of blood supply.

Heart failure: a weakened heart muscle that is unable to push blood forward

Heat cramps: painful muscle spasms due to excessive loss of fluid and salts by sweating.

Heat exhaustion: excessive sweating causing a loss of water and salts.

Heat stroke: a life-threatening emergency where the temperature regulation mechanism cannot cool the body and the temperature is far above normal.

Heimlich manoeuvre: abdominal thrusts done to remove an airway obstruction.

History: information about the casualty's problem: symptoms, events leading up to the problem, applicable illnesses or medications, etc.

Hyperglycemia: abnormally elevated blood sugar.

Hypertension: high blood pressure.

Hyperthermia: too high body temperature.

Hyperventilation: too deep and rapid respirations.

Hypoglycemia: too low blood sugar levels.

Hypothermia: too low body temperature.

Hypoxia: too low levels of oxygen in the body tissues.

I

Impaled object: an object which remains embedded in a wound.

Immobilization: placing some type of restraint along a body part to prevent movement.

Incontinence: loss of bladder and bowel control.

Infarction: an area of tissue death due to lack of blood flow.

Infection: inflammation due to microbes.

Inflammation: a tissue reaction to irritation, illness or injury; shows as redness, heat, swelling, and pain.

Inhalation: breathing in; inspiration.

Insulin: hormone produced by the pancreas; important in the regulation of blood sugar levels.

Insulin coma/reaction/shock: hypoglycemia (too low blood sugar levels) due to excessive insulin.

Intrapleural space: a tiny space containing a negative pressure (vacuum) between the two pleural layers.

Involuntary muscle: muscles not under conscious control; heart, intestines etc.

Iris: coloured part of the eye; made of muscles which control light entering the eye.

Ischemic: lacking sufficient oxygen; as in ischemic heart disease.

J

Joint: a place where two or more bones meet.

Joint capsule: a tough covering over a joint.

K

Kidneys: a pair of organs which filter blood and produce urine.

L

Labour: the muscular contractions of the uterus which expel the fetus.

Laceration: a jagged wound from a rip or a tear.

Laryngectomy: removal of the larynx (voice-box); results in a neck-breather.

Lens: a part of the eye which focuses light rays on the retina.

Ligament: a tough cord of tissue which connects bone to bone.

Lipoproteins: substances floating in the blood; made of proteins and fats.

Lymph: a fluid similar to plasma that circulates in the lymphatic system.

Lymphatic system: a system of vessels, nodes and organs which collects strayed proteins leaked from blood vessels and cleanses the body of microbes and other foreign matter.

M

Mandible: the bone of the lower jaw.

Mechanism of injury: the force that causes an injury and the way it is applied to the body.

Medical alert: a means of identifying casualties (usually a bracelet, necklace) who have a condition that may alter first aid treatment.

Medical help: the treatment given by or under the supervision of a medical doctor.

Mental Health Continuum: The Mental Health Continuum shows the range of mental health. Those with mental health illness or mental health problems can move through this range of healthy, reacting, injured and ill.

Mental Health Problem: A mental health problem is a broad term that includes both mental disorders and symptoms of mental disorders which may not be severe enough to warrant a diagnosis of a mental disorder.

Metacarpals: bones of the palm of the hand.

Metatarsals: bones of the arch of the foot; between the ankle and toes.

Micro-organisms: germs which can cause illness.

Miscarriage: the lay term for an abortion; the loss of the products of conception.

Mouth-to-mouth ventilation: artificial respiration by blowing air into the mouth of the casualty.

Mucous membrane: thin, slick, transparent lining, covering tubes and cavities that open to the outside; the inner surface of the mouth, nose, eye, ear, rectum, etc.

Musculoskeletal system: all of the bones, muscles, and connecting tissues which allow locomotion (movement of the body).

Myocardial infarction: death of part of the cardiac (heart) muscle; heart attack.

N

Nail bed test: a method of assessing the adequacy of circulation to the extremities; gentle pressure is exerted on the nail bed until the tissue whitens; the return of colour to the area is assessed upon pressure release.

Negligence: failure to perform first aid at the level expected of someone with similar training and experience.

Nerve: a cord made up of fibres which carry nerve impulses to and from the brain.

Nervous system: the brain, spinal cord and nerves which control the body's activities.

Nitroglycerin: a drug used to ease the workload on the heart; often carried as a pill or spray by casualties with angina.

O

O_2: the chemical symbol for oxygen.

Obstructed airway: a blockage in the air passageway to the lungs.

Oxygen: an odourless, colourless gas essential to life.

P

Pancreas: an organ located under the stomach; produces digestive enzymes and hormones which regulate blood sugar.

Paralysis: the loss of muscle function in part of the body.

Patella: the bone of the knee cap.

Phalanges: bones of the fingers and toes.

Pharynx: the back of the mouth and above the voice box (larynx); a passageway for both air and food.

Physiology: the study of functions of the body.

Placenta: an organ attached to the uterus which provides a fetus with nourishment.

Plasma: a pale yellow fluid containing blood cells, nutrients, gases and hormones.

Platelet: a small, cell-like blood element important in blood clotting.

G

Pleural membrane: a slick membrane covering the outside surface of the lungs and the inside surface of the chest cavity (thorax).

Pneumonia: inflammation of the lungs.

Pneumothorax: an accumulation of air in the pleural space. Normally the pleural space contains a negative pressure or a vacuum; the air mass (instead of a vacuum) collapses the lung under it.

Position of function: refers to the position an injured hand is placed in when bandaged and/or splinted; i.e. fingers are gently curved with palm slightly downwards.

Primary survey: a step of ESM—assessing the casualty for life-threatening injuries and giving appropriate first aid.

Proximal: refers to a part that is closest to the attachment of a leg/arm/finger/toe/intestine.

Pulmonary artery: the major artery emerging from the right ventricle; carries deoxygenated blood to the lungs.

Pulse: the rhythmic expansion and relaxation of the arteries caused by the contractile force of the heart; usually felt where the vessels cross a bone near the surface.

R

Radiate: to diverge or spread from a common point; the pain of a heart attack in the chest radiates to the left arm.

Radius: the bone on the thumb side of the lower arm.

Red blood cells: the most numerous type of blood cells; carry oxygen.

Respiratory arrest: stopped breathing.

Retina: the covering at the back of the eyeball; changes light rays into nerve impulses.

Reye's Syndrome: A rare but serious disease in children and adolescents that is reported to be associated with taking ASA for a viral infection. Reye's Syndrome affects the brain, liver and blood. It can cause permanent brain damage or death.

RICE.: R=rest; I= Immobilize; C= Cold; E= elevation. First aid for certain bone and joint injuries.

Rule of nines: a system of estimating the amount of skin surface burned.

S

Sacrum: a bone formed from five fused vertebra; forms the back of the pelvis.

Scapula: shoulder blade.

Scene survey: the initial step of ESM (emergency scene management) where the first aider takes control, assesses any hazards and makes the area safe, finds out what has happened, identifies self as a first aider, gains consent from the casualty, calls for help from bystanders and starts organizing them to get help for the casualty.

Sclera: the white of the eye; the tough, opaque layer of the eyeball.

Secondary survey: a step of ESM; assessing the casualty for non-life-threatening injuries and giving appropriate first aid.

Sign: objective evidence of disease or injury.

Sling: a support for an arm or shoulder, usually brought around the neck.

Spleen: an organ of the lymphatic system; functions to cleanse foreign matter from the blood; blood reservoir.

Spontaneous pneumothorax: air in the pleural space due to an unexplained rupture of the underlying lung.

Splint: is a rigid and padded support used to prevent movement in a bone or joint injury.

Sprain: supporting tissues about a joint (such as ligaments) are stretched, partly or completely torn.

Sternum: the breastbone.

Stoma: an opening in the neck through which the person breathes.

Strain: a stretched or torn muscle.

Sucking chest wound: a wound in which air is pulled into the chest cavity through the chest wall; it can cause a collapse of the lung beneath.

Superficial: on the surface of the body; as opposed to deep.

Superior vena cava: one of the two largest veins; it drains the arms and head of deoxygenated blood and empties into the right atrium.

Symptom: an indication of illness or injury experienced by a casualty; cannot be detected by an observer without asking.

Syrup of ipecac: an emetic; used to cause vomiting.

T

Tendon: a tough cord of tissue that attaches muscles to bones or other tissues.

Tension pneumothorax: air in the pleural space presses on the heart and blood vessels and affects their function.

Tetanus: a type of bacteria in a wound; can cause severe muscle spasms.

TIA: **transient ischemic attack**: a mini-stroke.

Tibia: the bone in the lower leg; on the large toe side; the shin bone.

Tonic phase: first stage of a convulsion where the muscles are rigid.

Tourniquet: a constricting band used to stop severe bleeding.

Trachea: a tube for air, kept open with cartilage rings; is located between the larynx (voice-box) and the bronchi.

Traction: gently but firmly pulling below a fracture to bring the limb into alignment.

Transient ischemic attack (TIA): temporary signs and symptoms of a stroke due to a lack of sufficient oxygen to the brain.

Trauma: any physical or psychological injury.

Triage: a system of placing priorities for first aid and/or transportation for multiple casualties.

U

Ulna: bone in the lower arm; on the little finger side.

Urethra: a tube which carries urine from the bladder to the outside.

Uterus: the muscular sac which holds, protects a fetus.

V

Vein: a blood vessel; carries blood to the heart.

Ventilation: supplying air to the lungs.

Ventricles: the muscular lower chambers of the heart which pump blood into the arteries.

Ventricular fibrillation: a quivering action of the heart muscles so that little blood is pumped.

Vital signs: the four signs that show the basic condition of the casualty: level of consciousness; breathing; pulse; skin condition and temperature (sources vary as to the components of vital signs).

W

White blood cells: blood cells which are involved in immunity and control of microbes.

X

Xiphoid process: the cartilage tip at the lower end of the breastbone.

G

Index

I

I

I

I

I